First-time parent

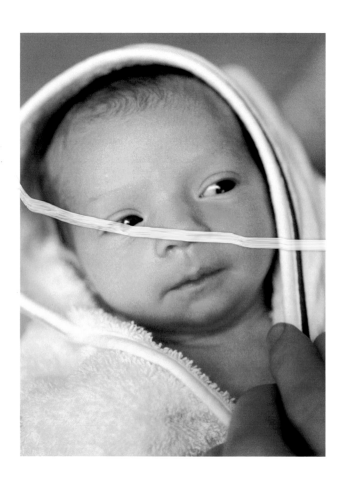

First-time parent

LUCY ATKINS

Collins

This paperback edition published in 2009 by Collins
an imprint of HarperCollins
77-85 Fulham Palace Road
London W6 8JB
www.collins.co.uk

Collins is a registered trademark of HarperCollins Publishers Ltd

10 9 8 7 6 5

Editor: Adam Parfitt
Photographer: Ben Cowlin
Design: Valle Walkley

A catalogue record for this book is available from the British Library

ISBN 978 0 00 726944 0

Printed and bound at Printing Express, Hong Kong

To my marvellous parents, with love and undying gratitude

contents

introduction

When I was pregnant for the first time, I found I had strong views on parenting that covered everything from what a wonderful, tolerant and inspired mother I would be, to how I would never, ever fill my house with all that depressing, tasteless baby gear. I am now a mother of three (aged six, four and one). Far from being inspired or in control, I generally feel I am living under the occupation of a force far, far greater than myself. I have, at various points in the past six years, been the owner of no less than eleven pushchairs. And my house looks like the inside of Toys 'R' Us. Parenthood for me – and I know I'm not alone here – is nothing like the books and magazines say it should be, and nothing like I thought it would be. It's far harder. Significantly less 'controllable'. And – thank God – infinitely more amazing.

My babies have had me sobbing with joy and despair. They've driven me to extremes of pleasure and boredom, anger and elation, pride and self-doubt. Nothing can really prepare you for all this first time around. But on a practical level, a few realistic pointers are certainly handy. And that's where this book comes in.

I'm not covering pregnancy or birth here – you can learn about that more fully, and usefully, elsewhere. Instead, this book gives you all the basics that you need to know about your baby's first year, starting with a shopping list (what do you really need, and what's just pointless?), and moving swiftly on to the moment your baby takes his first breath. You'll then learn about the feeds – How often? How much? How long? How on earth??? – the crying, the sleeping, poos, burps, farts, common illnesses and developmental milestones of your baby's first year.

Above all, though, this book is designed to keep you sane. Yes, you need to know what to do if your baby's poo turns green; but you also need to know that feeling incompetent, confused or just plain crackers is an entirely normal and understandable part of parenthood. One, in my view, that's largely ignored by baby books.

Once you have a baby, the world certainly does change. Indeed, the whole notion of 'love' takes on a new and extraordinary significance when you become a parent. But this does not mean you have turned into a completely different person. You don't start wearing disgraceful leggings and enormous yellow T-shirts just because you're a new parent. Nor do you lose all your other critical faculties. And this book reflects that. You may now be bonkers, but you're not stupid. So trust yourself: though sleep-deprived and covered in baby sick, in your infant's eyes at least, you're the only expert that matters.

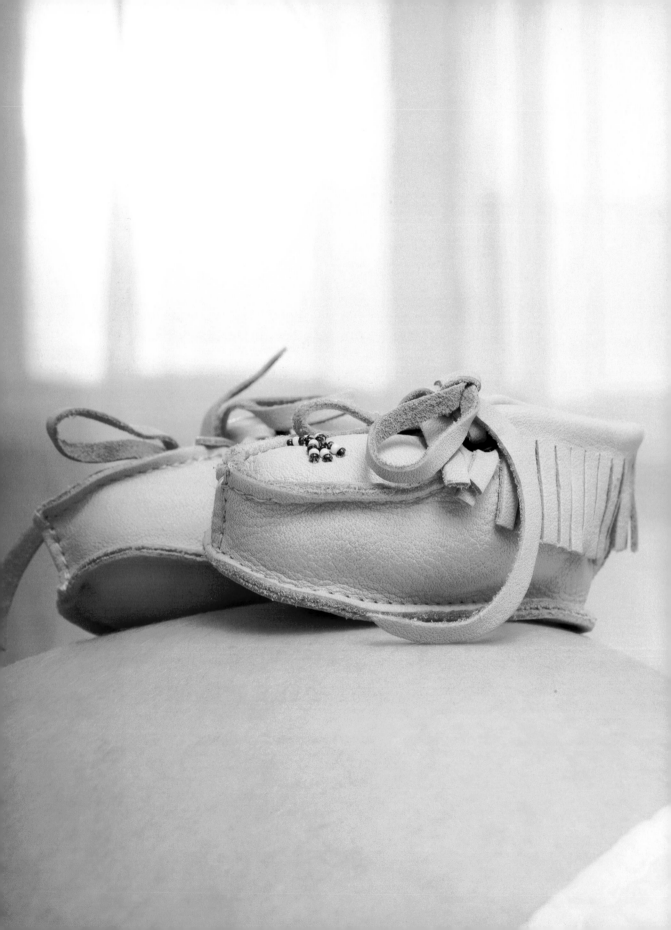

prepare

The stuff you need, and the stuff you don't ...

Clearly nothing can really prepare you for parenthood, but most of us don't need any encouragement when let loose in the baby section of a department store. There are plenty of fabulous accessories and gizmos for you to spend your money on. But actually, babies have extremely basic requirements. They need somewhere to sleep, some sort of transport for outings, some clothes and nappies and things to wipe their bottoms with. And milk. And you.

Essential clothes

As far as clothes are concerned, keep it simple. Buy soft, stretchy, cotton clothes as you want dressing to be as quick and painless as possible. Babygros that have poppers (or a zip) from neck to crotch and down the legs are easiest. Buttons and poppers that go up the back are a pain in the neck and any 'little adult' type clothes – jeans, button-up shirts, jackets and the like – are just silly for little babies: they are uncomfortable (imagine if YOU had to sleep in them), not stretchy enough to allow free movement, and are soon outgrown.

THE MINIMUM YOU'LL NEED TO GET YOUR BABY
THROUGH THE FIRST MONTH OR SO IS:

- Six cotton vests (long or short sleeved depending on season)
- Six to ten cotton Babygros
- Six pairs of socks (stretchy towelling ones tend to stay on better – booties are generally pointless as they fall off teeny feet)
- Two to three cardigans (easier than jumpers)
- A couple of cotton hats
- A warm, all-in-one, padded suit for outings if you have a winter baby

For the first few weeks, your baby will practically live in Babygros.

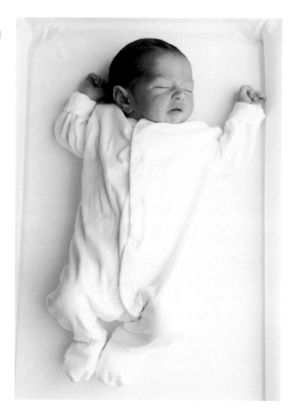

Borrow stuff if you can, or buy second-hand: babies grow out of things in seconds. Try the NCT's 'nearly new' sales, eBay, your local newspaper, charity shops, jumble sales and school fêtes. Accept all offers of hand-me-downs from friends with bigger kids.

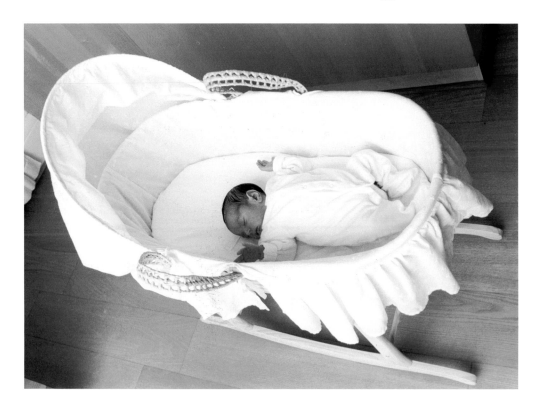

Essential equipment

Aside from clothes, there are a few other essentials that you should try to buy before the baby arrives:

- At least four packs of newborn nappies (if you are using disposables). Take a pack to the hospital. You'll change a newborn's nappy about sixty times a week at the start.
- Three large rolls of cotton wool for wiping bottoms and washing generally
- A pack of (unperfumed) baby wipes for outings – it's hard to do the cotton-wool-and-water bottom-wiping thing in, say, a park
- A car seat suitable from birth *(see page 21)*
- A buggy *(see page 18)*
- A crib or Moses basket with a mattress that's British Safety Standard certified. Most babies don't go in a bigger cot until they're three to five months old.

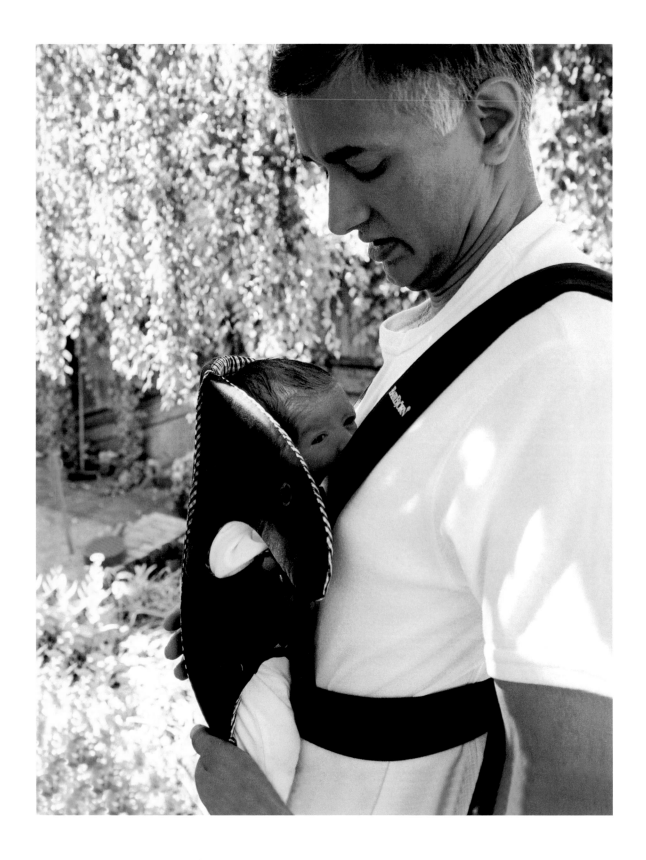

- Three or four cot sheets and a Grobag baby sleeping bag appropriate for the season and your baby's size, or three to four cellular blankets. Never use duvets or quilts with babies under one because they can overheat. Most experienced parents will tell you that buying a Grobag was the best thing they ever did. It stops your baby kicking off the covers and waking (you!) up because he's cold.
- About ten muslin squares (get them in packs from Mothercare or Boots) for wiping up baby sick, protecting your clothes from dribble, lying the baby on in a park or making an impromptu sun hat – or, indeed, an 'I surrender' flag.

Other useful, but not totally essential, baby equipment

This is stuff you don't *have* to get, but if you do it could make your life a hell of a lot easier:

- A baby monitor – this way you can hear your baby wherever you are in the house or garden. Basic models are fine.
- A bouncy sling-type chair to sit him safely in when he is awake
- A baby-carrying sling – good for fussy or colicky babies, or for just getting around when he's small enough to be easily portable. My Baby Björn sling lasted through three babies and is now being used by a friend.
- A fleece or soft, thick rug to lie your baby on when he's awake and needs to kick around a bit
- A wipe-down nappy-changing mat (or you can just use an old towel)
- A nappy bag (discuss whether you both really want the one with pink teddy logos) with travel changing mat. It doesn't have to be a specific 'nappy' bag – you can use any bag at all, as long as it is big enough to fit:

  - Three or four nappies
  - A pack of wipes
  - A small, folding changing mat
  - A small pot of nappy-rash cream
  - A complete change of baby clothing
  - A toy or two, and maybe a book for you
  - A water bottle and maybe a snack for you
  - A baby-feeding bottle and small carton of formula if bottle-feeding
  - Your phone, wallet and keys

Postnatal shopping list

FOR YOUR VAGINA/PERINEUM

● = BASICS
(if nothing else, get these)

- Several small packets of frozen peas to soothe your perineum
- Squeezy bottles or jugs for pouring on yourself as you pee *(see page 38)*
- Large cotton-feel sanitary pads or 'maternity' pads
- Disposable or old/cheapo knickers (ten to fifteen pairs). Bin them when messy.
- A couple of pairs of comfy pyjamas that fit you when pregnant
- A bottle of witch hazel for soothing your sore bits *(see page 40)*
- A sitz bath (or plastic basin) you can use to bathe your bits after vaginal birth, plus essential oils or herbs to add *(see page 39)*

FOR YOUR BREASTFEEDING BOOBS

- Two or three soft breastfeeding bras
- The telephone number of your hospital's infant-feeding specialist and other breastfeeding counsellors
- Several packets of breast pads to stop your breasts leaking on to your shirt
- Extra pillows – good for propping up the baby while breastfeeding
- A footstool to help with a good breastfeeding position (a few old phone directories taped together with masking tape work fine)
- Lanisoh for sore nipples. You can buy this in Waitrose and some chemists.
- A breast pump

GENERALLY

- A large pack of paracetamol (for afterpains)
- A hot water bottle (ditto)
- Lots of healthy meals for your freezer (such as portions of home-made soup, casseroles and pasta sauces)
- Soft stretchy clothes like sweatpants
- Any midwife-recommended postnatal vitamins and iron tablets

Feeding equipment

IF BREASTFEEDING (WHOEVER SAID IT WAS 'FREE'?)

- Your boobs (any size and shape will do)
- Three comfy but oh-so-stylish feeding bras (Elle Macpherson does a fantastic range available from www.bloomingmarvellous.com)
- Breastfeeding help numbers (see **Contacts**), including your hospital breastfeeding specialist if there is one
- A breast pump. Manual pumps are generally cheaper, quieter and more portable than electric ones, but they can be hard work and slow. Electrics tend to be faster and, for some, more effective. You can hire a breast pump from the NCT, or you can borrow one from your hospital's breastfeeding clinic. Two good ones are the Medela Harmony Mini Electric (www.medela.co.uk) and the Avent Isis Manual (www.avent.com).
- Pre-sterilised bags are useful for storing breast milk if you are breastfeeding and want to pump and freeze milk to feed your baby in a bottle sometimes.

IF BOTTLE-FEEDING

- About six 250–280 ml bottles, with 'slow flow' newborn teats to start with. There are all sorts of bottles on the market, but both Avent and Boots own brand are perfectly good ones to start with.
- A way to sterilise them *(see page 112)*
- A baby-bottle brush for washing them up
- A supply of powdered baby formula. Most infant formula milks are based on modified cow's milk. If you think your baby may be allergic to cow's milk, talk to your GP – don't buy over-the-counter alternatives like soya or goat's milk as they may make your baby ill. SMA is a well-known brand of formula, and Hipp Organics does a popular (if pricey) organic formula available in many supermarkets (and Boots).
- Cartons of formula for feeding on the go

What buggy?

'Buggy', 'stroller', 'pushchair', 'pram', 'three-in-one', 'travel system', 'jogger': there are countless devices for transporting your baby from A to B. In essence, you need to buy some form of transport for your newborn that lies flat for the first three months, because tiny babies don't have the head control to cope with sitting more upright. After about three months you want to be able to raise the back of the buggy seat up progressively so that, by about six months, your baby can sit up in it. You can buy expensive lie-flat prams for new babies, but they'll be redundant after a few months. As a basic rule, if you want a buggy to last you from birth to four years, it needs to be lightweight, easily foldable and have a back that can lie flat but with several more upright positions too.

You can buy 'travel systems' or 'three-in-ones', which give you an infant car seat, pram and pushchair in one package. If you get one of these, make it lightweight or you'll almost certainly ditch it when your baby reaches about six months, as it'll become too clumsy and hefty. After about six months a lightweight 'umbrella-type' stroller that folds easily is really all you need (you can buy these suitable from birth – Maclaren does a popular one that lies flat for newborns).

As for the rest, in general, buggy accessories add money but not much value. The only really useful 'extras' are: somewhere to put your shopping (a sling-type pocket under the buggy is fine); a good rain cover; some form of sun canopy (you can buy clip-on sun umbrellas) and, in the winter, a 'cosy toes' sleeping bag that fits on the buggy can be handy (blankets slip off easily when you're mobile).

WHEN CHOOSING YOUR BUGGY, YOU SHOULD ALSO CONSIDER:

- What you'll use it for. Will it fit in your front door and into your car? Will you be mostly in the city or jogging down country lanes? Carrying it up stairs? On to buses?
- How long you want it to last. The first few months? Or all the way to three or four years?
- Your budget. But bear in mind that cheapo ones can be a false economy – they break, or you just get sick to death of how crap they are then crack and buy a pricey one.
- Quality. Forget the fabric design – you want it to be easy to steer, solid, relatively lightweight, reasonably padded with good suspension and a smooth folding action.

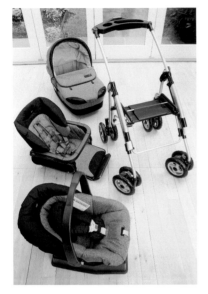

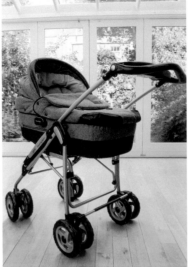

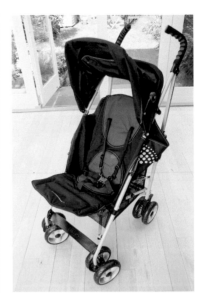

The constituent parts of a 'three-in-one' (clockwise from bottom): the car seat, the buggy fitting (which can lie flat or upright), the carry cot and the frame. *(above)*

You can fit the carry cot, the car seat or the buggy fitting on to the basic frame.

From about six months you'll probably decide to ditch this stuff and get a lightweight 'umbrella-type' stroller. *(right)*

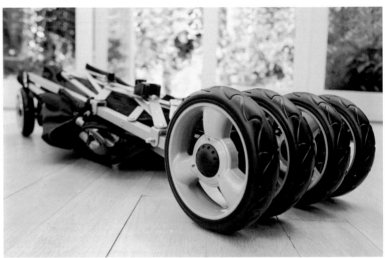

For details of all these companies, see **Contacts**.

Mamas & Papas, my favourite, do lightweight buggies that lie completely flat for a newborn but work all the way to four. Babydan are sturdy and Graco are lower budget but OK. For a posh long-lasting three-wheeler (from New Zealand, home of outdoorsy fanatics) try Phil & Ted's. Bugaboo is the latest trendy design with great features. For double buggies, Mountain Buggy Urban Double is a top-of-the-range three-wheeler from birth to four years, and Maclaren do a popular, solid but not heavy 'umbrella' double buggy.

Go and try out a display model in Mothercare or Babies 'R' Us before you buy it at half the price online. A great place for baby equipment is eBay.

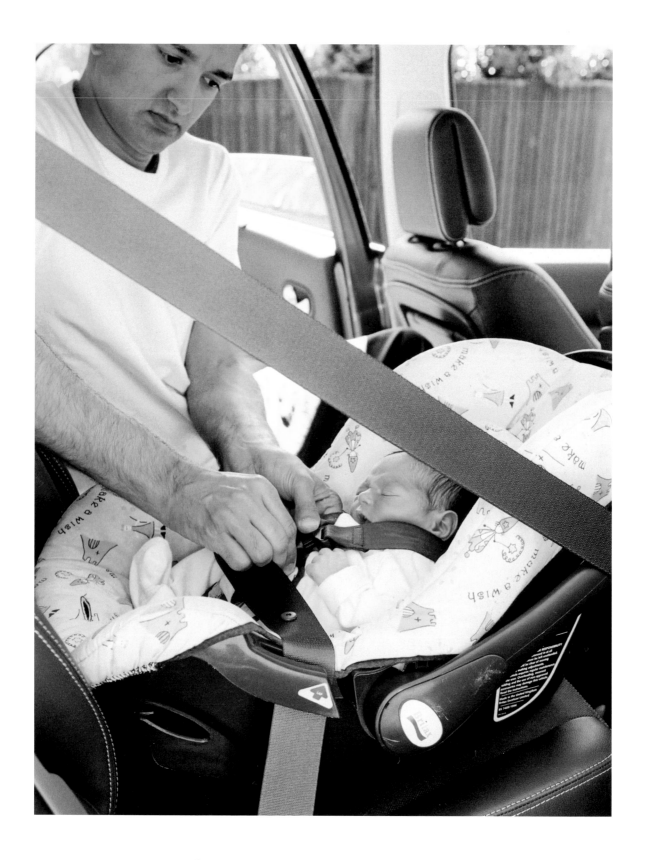

What car seat?

Car accidents are a leading cause of death and injury in children, so this is one to take very, very seriously. You can buy car seats suitable from birth to four years, or a backwards-facing baby seat suitable until nine to twelve months (depending on the size of your baby), then a car seat suitable from about nine months to four years. The backwards-facing baby seat is useful as you can clip it in and out of the car and carry or sit your baby in it when you're in cafés or friends' houses.

THERE ARE CERTAIN CAR-SAFETY RULES YOU SHOULD *ALWAYS* FOLLOW:

- Always put your baby in a properly fitted seat, suitable for his age and weight.
- Be sure the car seat is genuinely a safe one. It should have a British Standard Kitemark or United Nations Standard Regulation 44.03 and is the one piece of equipment you shouldn't buy second-hand unless you know its history (i.e. no accidents) and have the instructions. For information on choosing the right car seat and fitting it correctly go to www.thinkroadsafety.gov.uk or www.childcarseats.org.uk.
- Never fit an infant car seat in the front seat of a car with air bags. The back seat is the safest place (unless your car is, freakishly, without back-seat seatbelts).
- Never *ever* take your baby out of the car seat when the car is moving, even if he is purple in the face and bellowing and your pulse is racing. We have all been tempted to do this but it's extremely dangerous. Always pull over somewhere safe before you get him out.

It is *essential* to have the correct car seat *(left)*. This is a backwards-facing baby seat suitable until nine to twelve months.

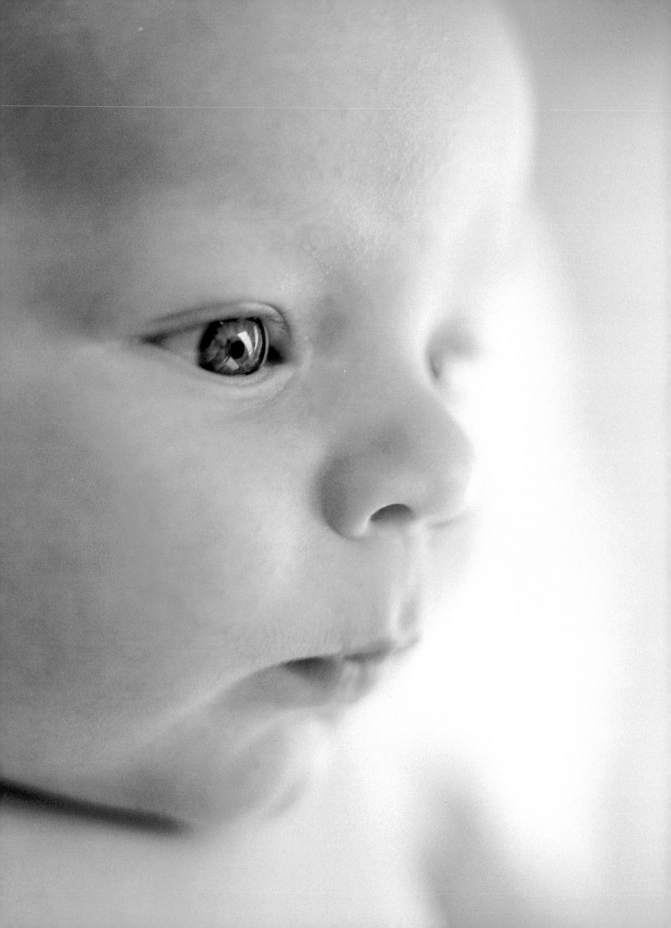

hello!

The mind-blowing first few days

For many of us, the first 'hello' is not as we'd expected. There is no lightening-strike recognition, no heavenly choir, no soft-focus twinning of souls. Most of us, after giving birth for the first time, are exhausted, shocked and mind-blown by the whole experience. And most new fathers are reeling too. That it can take a while for 'baby love' to kick in (and it will, eventually) says nothing about your capacity to be the world's greatest parent. Meeting your new baby can truly be the best moment of your life. But equally, it can be a bit weird.

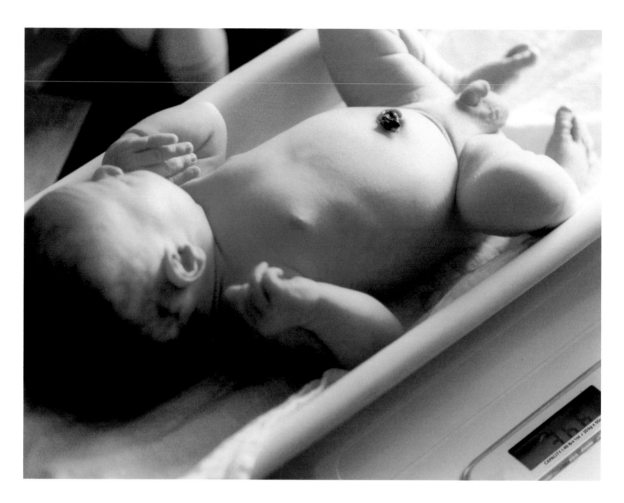

What happens immediately after the birth?

Head, shoulders, body … a rush of fluids and astonishment: you've done it! It's a real baby, right there, and she's *yours*. Your baby should – the moment she's out – be put on to your tummy with her skin against your skin ('skin to skin'), usually with a towel over her to keep her warm. She does not need to be whisked off to be washed, weighed, measured or anything else at this point, unless she needs urgent medical attention, in which case she will be taken to a resuscitation area in the delivery room where the doctor will help her. But if all is well, your baby belongs on you and you alone now, and if possible you want to keep her there, skin to skin, for at least the first thirty minutes of her life. Studies show this really helps mother–baby bonding, reduces crying and helps breastfeeding. It's really worth putting this in your birth plan as it may not automatically happen.

If you have a Caesarean and your baby doesn't need urgent medical attention, ask to have her put immediately on your chest against your skin, lying across your body with your partner's hand supporting her back or bottom. If she is healthy there's every reason to keep your baby as close to you as you would after a vaginal birth. You may get knee-jerk objections to this from staff who have never been asked to do it before. But it is your baby, so be assertive.

After a vaginal birth, if the midwife speeds up the delivery of your placenta with an injection (a 'managed third stage'), she'll cut the umbilical cord as soon as your baby emerges. But if you have chosen to deliver the placenta without an injection, the midwife will leave the cord until it stops pulsing. This isn't as freaky as it sounds: blood rich in oxygen and nutrients carries on going into your baby via the cord for a short while after she is born. Sometimes the cord does not stop delivering this blood to your baby until after the placenta is out. Many dads decide to take the scissors for this historic cord-cutting moment, and it is completely trauma-free: the cord has no nerves, so cutting it is painless for mother and baby, and there is no blood. The midwife then clamps the end of the cord with a plastic clip near your baby's tummy. This 'stump' will drop off some time in the next two weeks, leaving a perfectly formed belly button.

THE **APGAR** SCORE DECODED

ACTIVITY/muscle tone: limp/ no response/active/taut arms and legs

PULSE/heart rate: absent to more than 100 beats per minute

GRIMACE: first breath response – none to sneeze or cough

APPEARANCE: colour – white/ blue/grey to pink all over

RESPIRATION: (absent to good/cry)

When your baby is only one minute old, the midwife or doctor will run down a quick 'healthy signs' checklist (in their head). They check your baby for five signs that she is healthy, and for each one they give her a score – anything from zero (bad) to two (the best possible). If, for instance, your baby has completely limp arms and legs, she'll get zero for 'Activity'. If she is moving a bit she'll get a one, and if she's actively wriggling – the healthiest sign in a newborn – she'll get a two. This score helps them to assess how well she has coped with the birth, and whether she needs any medical attention. The most a baby can get is a ten, though it's rare to get this at one minute. By five minutes, when the Apgar score is done again, most babies are a good solid ten.

How soon your baby will want a feed after the birth varies, but if you are both healthy, the midwife should help you to try your first breastfeed within about thirty minutes of giving birth.

After the birth you will usually stay put in your delivery suite for a couple of hours. If you tore or had an episiotomy, the midwife or doctor will stitch you up; she'll also weigh your baby, and put two identity tags on each of her ankles. You should be offered the chance to pee, have a shower or wash. It's absolutely fine to have a bath at any point after giving birth, but don't make it too hot or you might faint – largely through exhaustion. Finally, after a couple of hours, when the midwife has done the paperwork, you have decided to name your baby after her and you are really, completely sure you've counted all those fingers and toes, you will be trundled on to the ward, usually in a wheelchair. You may be allowed to carry your baby in your arms as you go, or it may be the hospital's policy to wheel your baby next to you in a Perspex cot (a see-through plastic box on trolley wheels that looks a bit like a prop in a 1960s B-movie). If the hospital insists on moving your baby in the cot and not in your arms, it is a health and safety thing: some units don't want to be put in a tricky position by exhausted mummies dropping babies en route to the ward.

If you had a Caesarean, you will be taken from the operating theatre into a recovery room or observation area. How long you stay in recovery varies from hospital to hospital. In some, you stay there for twelve to twenty-four hours; in others, you'll only be there for a couple of hours before being taken to the ward. But you'll be very closely monitored wherever you are for the first twenty-four hours after a surgical birth, and you'll need regular doses of pain relief.

Vitamin K

This makes our blood clot properly. On rare occasions, a newborn doesn't have enough and may bleed dangerously (known as 'vitamin K deficiency bleeding'). Most newborns now are given vitamin K by injection when they are first born, but you can give it orally in two doses when she's a few days old. Some studies in the 1990s raised worries about a link between injected vitamin K and childhood cancer, but the current scientific consensus is that there is no evidence to support these worries and that injected vitamin K is safe. Ideally this is something you should think about before the birth – talk to your midwife.

'Recovery'

After the midwife or doctor has made sure you and the baby are doing well, they'll leave you all together for a bit – possibly in a 'recovery room' – so that you can get to know one another, before moving you to the ward where a Perspex cot will be put next to your bed. It can be unsettling and even strangely lonely to find that you – and you alone – are suddenly in charge of your tiny newborn. Midwives may be too busy to answer questions like 'Am I holding her right?'.

Most new mothers, when they talk about the midwives they had for the birth, are overcome with gratitude and admiration. Midwives in general do a superlative job. But they are not superhuman. On the maternity ward the midwives are likely to be extremely over-stretched. 'There was one midwife for ten women on the ward,' says Heather. 'I had had a C-section and couldn't pick Ellie up to cuddle or feed her. At one point she was crying next to me for 40 minutes and the midwife couldn't help me pick her up because she was having to deal with other requests. This was awful – I eventually just burst into tears myself.' You may have to be very assertive to get attention and you will certainly have to wait unless it's an emergency. It's a good idea to call the midwife early if you have any inkling that you are going to need something (for instance, if you need help to go to the loo or are going to need painkillers soon).

If it is night-time, fathers are then sent home – no dads are allowed on the ward at night. This is why you want your partner there as much as possible during the day. 'I wasn't prepared for the first hours alone with the baby,' says Sara, mother of Tom, nine months. 'He was born in the early hours of the morning, and my partner and mum didn't pitch up again at hospital until the afternoon, which really upset me. I'd say company and support on day one is of paramount importance.' You may be discharged as little as six hours after an uncomplicated birth, but most of us leave hospital about twenty-four hours after giving birth vaginally and three to five days after a Caesarean. If there are any complications, you may have to stay longer.

YOU MIGHT WANT TO:

- Bring earplugs. Wards are noisy, and you can use them when your partner has the baby to get some uninterrupted sleep.
- Ask for what you need, no matter how frantic, brusque or irritated the midwives seem.
- Investigate the possibility of a single room: it costs anything from £30–£500 depending on your hospital, but having one means you get peace and quiet – and your partner can stay too.
- Prepare yourself to be really assertive when you need help from the midwife – at the very least with establishing feeding or if you think something may be wrong.
- Work out in advance who will visit you in hospital. You may not feel like greeting six of your work colleagues after a forty-eight-hour labour when you are attempting your first nappy change.

Dads, meanwhile, are left in an elated, buzzing state of limbo – and probably exhaustion. The really key thing to do, if you possibly can, is wind down a bit.

Dads: what else should you be doing?

When you are sent home, once you have stopped sobbing you could:

- Email family and friends: have a 'group' set up, and just fire off the baby-arrival message.
- Sleep – it's your one chance. There will be little of it when your baby gets home.
- Tidy up, so your partner does not come back to a bomb site.
- Fit the baby seat in the car and understand how to clip it in and out and buckle it up efficiently.
- Go to the shops: get basic supplies for home like bread and milk, and also *the biggest bunch of blooms you can get your hands on* (take to the hospital!) Hospital food is gruesome so take her some food too – a few treats, healthy snacks and even simple meals (fibre-rich foods like dried or soft fruit is good).
- Zoom back to the hospital – don't leave her alone with the baby for longer than absolutely necessary.

'And, most importantly, tell her – *repeatedly and grovellingly* – how proud you are of what she's just done.'

Back in the hospital, don't be afraid to take photos and video footage – these will be precious one day. And, most importantly, tell her – *repeatedly and grovellingly* – how proud you are of what she's just done. Whatever happened in that labour room – a planned Caesarean, drugs, tongs, suction devices, ten hours of her yelling abuse and battering you – at this point she needs to know you think she's amazing and that you love her more than ever before. Make this your fallback position for the coming months.

Special care

The best place to get more information and support on scbu is the charity bliss – see **Contacts** for details.

If your baby needs to go to the Special Care Baby Unit (scbu), perhaps because she is born early, is ill or has some health problem, it can be scary and upsetting to say the least. One in ten babies need special care at birth, and the vast majority are fine (forty per cent of twins and over ninety-seven per cent of triplets spend some time in special care). Many of these babies need to be in an incubator and fed through a tube until they're well enough to do it by themselves. There are a number of reasons why your baby might need special care:

BORN EARLY

Babies born before thirty-seven weeks' gestation are considered 'premature'. Some premature babies are fine, but if your baby is born at less than thirty-four weeks, she will almost certainly need to go to special care. Possible difficulties include not sucking properly, poor temperature control and immature lungs.

Babies born early haven't had time to put on weight like term babies, so can look a bit different. They may have loose, wrinkled, red skin, be covered in downy hair ('lanugo'), have a very big-looking head and skinny little body, have uneven or heavy breathing, and they might move very jerkily.

'It's important to remember that even though they look really scary, attached to wires, probes, drips and drains, they are still your little baby,' says Lisa Hynes. Her first baby, Milo (now six), spent several weeks in scbu, and her third baby, Lara (now eighteen months), spent six months in scbu. 'With Milo I was so scared of touching him – he would ping if moved – that I had to be encouraged to hold him as he seemed such a scary medical bundle. With Lara I was no longer scared of it all as I had seen it before and I understood the machinery. That made a big difference.'

LOW BIRTHWEIGHT

Some babies born after thirty-seven weeks are smaller than they should be and so have fewer fat stores. Your baby may be able to stay with you in the postnatal ward, but the doctors will probably need to do regular blood-sugar checks to monitor her progress. Possible difficulties include poor temperature control and trouble controlling the glucose supply in the blood.

INFECTION

Infections in newborn babies have numerous causes and often very non-specific symptoms, which is why paediatricians tend to prescribe antibiotics just in case. Usually it takes about forty-eight hours to get test results to show what, if anything, is causing any infection.

OTHER HEALTH RISKS

A baby who had difficulties breathing at birth or has a known birth defect, like a 'hole in the heart', or who is jaundiced *(see page 32)* may need special care.

Ways to cope with SCBU

- Ask for information, no matter how busy and cross the staff look.
- Take breaks. Getting away for a walk or a bite to eat with your partner is crucial: scbu is emotionally draining.
- Remember it's *your* baby. You can help care for her through this – ask staff to show you what you can do.
- Don't give up on bonding. Staff can show you how to touch and comfort your baby even when she's in an incubator (she'll recognise your voice and smell). Any skin-to-skin contact you can have is very valuable.
- Understand the monitors: they are very sensitive and alarms tend to go off regularly. If you understand what they mean, you'll feel less stressed.
- Get clear feedback. If your baby has a setback, ask your doctor to rate it on a scale of one to ten. This will help you get a handle on how serious it is.
- Be sensitive to others. Babies arrive all the time, so try to give other families privacy and train your visitors to observe the rules in scbu.
- Don't give up on breastfeeding. Ask to see the hospital's breast-feeding specialist and get her to show you exactly how – and how often – to use the breast pump so you can still feed your baby.
- Visit your baby whenever you want. 'scbu is open twenty-four hours a day,' says Lisa Hynes. 'If you are still in hospital and you wake up at 3 a.m. and want to see your baby, then go and sit with her, stroke her head, do whatever you can do that makes you feel better. The nurses can be quite hostile or surprised at that time of the night, but I felt so strongly that they were my babies and if I were feeding them I would be up anyway. At night you feel the separation from the baby most keenly, so if you want to see them, stuff the frowning looks and go.'

Your new baby

What newborns do

In the first twenty-four hours, most babies (though by no means all) tend to sleep most of the time. But she'll also wake up from time to time and want to feel you there, touching, holding, cuddling and feeding her. She may look like she's in a world of her own, but actually she's totally wired up to you:

- She can see your face clearly if it's 20-25 cm (8-10 in) from hers, will respond with a raised heart rate when she does, and will probably make eye contact. She may even mirror your facial movements – try sticking out your tongue at her.
- She can recognise her parents' voices.
- She can probably recognise her mother's smell.
- She has an inbuilt set of reflexes. She'll:

  ⟶ grasp anything put into her fist
  ⟶ suck and swallow
  ⟶ take a 'step' if you hold her up with toes touching a surface
  ⟶ 'startle' (the 'Moro reflex'). If she hears a loud noise, she will throw her arms up suddenly, as if stopping herself from falling.
  ⟶ root for the nipple. If you stroke her cheek with your finger or breast, she'll turn her head, looking for the nipple.

Yes, she really can see you! From a distance of 20-25 cm your newborn focuses clearly.

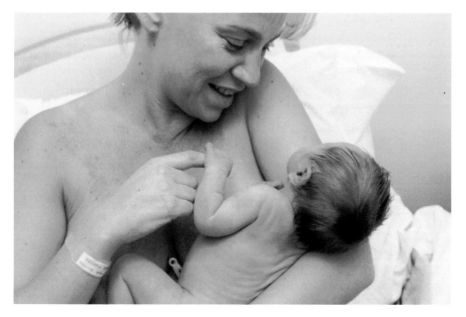

What newborns look like

Being born is no picnic, so don't expect to see a perfectly formed little beauty at first. Newborns often have a puffy, boxer-type face, and many have temporarily 'cone-shaped' heads from the journey out. If the birth involved a ventouse (a suction device), the top of your baby's head may bulge noticeably and have a circular red mark on it. Similarly a forceps-delivered baby may have temporary marks where the tongs were. Caesarean-born babies, particularly if the Caesarean was planned, tend to be more 'perfect' looking.

A 'term' baby (one not born prematurely) can be anything from 5 lb to a whopping 10 lb or more. Twins on average weigh 5 lb 8 oz, but it's normal for one twin to be much bigger than the other.

'Being born is no picnic, so don't expect to see a perfectly formed little beauty at first.'

A greyish-blue colour at birth is normal (even with black or Asian babies, which has thrown many an unsuspecting dad), but within a few breaths they generally turn a more 'healthy' colour. Their skin can stay red, blotchy, peely, flaky or significantly lighter or darker than you'd expect for a while though. Some babies are also born covered in vernix (white, creamy stuff that protects their skin in the womb: you don't need to wipe this off – it's good for the baby's skin).

Birthmarks are common, harmless and usually temporary. A 'stork mark' at the nape of the neck or eyelids caused by dilated blood vessels is the most common; it generally disappears within the first year. 'Strawberry' birthmarks – raised and red with a dotted effect – appear in about ten per cent of babies within four weeks and usually fade within two years. 'Port-wine stain' birthmarks are flat, red marks found in about 2 in 1,000 babies and don't usually fade away. Ask your midwife if you have any birthmark concerns.

If the whites of your baby's eyes and the skin below her nipple line are turning yellowish, it may be jaundice. Jaundice can be caused by prematurity, bruising at birth, infection or exposure to drugs the mother may have had in labour. Most newborns will become a little bit jaundiced between day two and day seven, and you should mention this to the midwife or GP if you notice it. Frequent feeding is usually recommended. Jaundice in the first forty-eight hours, however, can be quite serious, so call the midwife or GP straight away if you notice anything amiss.

If the midwife thinks your baby is jaundiced, she may take some blood from your baby's heel. This helps her to work out how jaundiced she is, and your baby may then need to be put under blue lights ('phototherapy') to clear it up. You may have to stay in hospital for a few days if this happens.

Another new-parent surprise is that newborn boys and girls often have swollen genitals and breasts. A tiny amount of milky discharge may come out of the nipples, and girl babies may even have a bit of bloody discharge from their vaginas. This is all caused by the mother's hormones circulating through the baby at birth; it is totally healthy and stops after a day or so.

Other surprises

In the first twenty-four to forty-eight hours, sticky secretions that your baby has swallowed during the birth can get stuck in her throat, making her choke and sometimes turn blue. If this happens, put her over your knee, face down, and give her a firm slap between the shoulders to clear the airways. If this doesn't work straight away, call for help. Some babies vomit up a bit of mucus spontaneously. Again, all this is completely normal, but scary if you don't know what to do.

Meanwhile, at the other end, your baby's first couple of poos will be a tar-like, sticky, greenish-black colour. This is meconium, the waste products she has accumulated in the womb. Most babies (ninety-four per cent) will pass meconium within twenty-four hours. But two to four per cent of normal babies don't pass meconium by forty-eight hours. If your baby has not done a black poo after about twenty-four hours, tell the midwife. If your baby is vomiting, or has a very tight, swollen belly and has not passed meconium, tell the doctor or midwife immediately.

BEFORE YOU TAKE YOUR BABY HOME, A DOCTOR WILL CHECK YOUR BABY'S:

- **Vision and hearing (a hearing test may be done by a special nurse)**
- **Heart and lungs**
- **Sucking reflex**
- **Internal organs**
- **Spine**
- **Hips**

Looking after your brand-new baby

All being well, all you'll have to do in the first forty-eight hours or so of your baby's life is feed, cuddle endlessly, change the odd nappy and take tons of photos. What could be simpler?

Cuddling

Studies have shown that skin-to-skin contact is important for parents and babies alike – it can help you bond with your baby and can help establish breastfeeding. Don't be afraid to open the poppers of her

Babygro and put her against your chest (dads too) to calm her down if she's yelling. Many newborns will only be content when cuddled close (if she can hear your heart beat she may be calmer), so don't feel she needs to be in that Perspex cot.

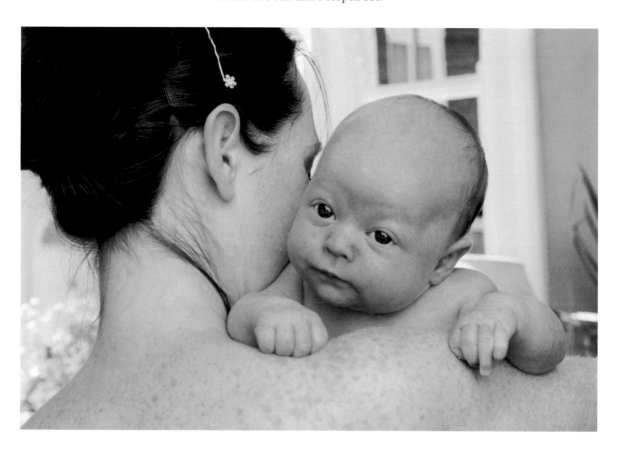

For everything you need to know about breast- or bottle-feeding from the first feed onwards, turn to **Chapter Six**.

Breastfeeding

If you're breastfeeding, your baby might want to latch on within as little as ten minutes of being born. Or it may take her a few more hours to get round to it.

SOME TIPS FOR THE FIRST FEED:

- Draw the curtains round your hospital bed so it's a bit quieter and less distracting for you both.
- Talk or sing to her – she'll be reassured by your voice.
- If she's crying, try to calm her by jiggling or soothing her. If she's in a lather it may be harder to get her to work out that it's a feed she wants.
- If you can't calm her, just offer her the breast or bottle.

Changing nappies

TIPS

- Never flush a nappy down the loo.

- Always wipe a girl baby from front to back (towards her bottom), and don't clean inside her labia.

- Wipe a boy baby all over his penis, testicles and bottom, but never pull back his foreskin to clean under it. Also, gently hold his penis down or you'll get an eyeful of pee.

- Often babies poo just as you've whipped the nappy away (or put a clean one on). Just keep on wiping.

- If you're using real nappies, follow the instructions they come with. If I were you I'd do a practice run with a baby doll before the birth.

- Bring to the hospital: cotton wool, newborn nappies and several Babygros. Unless there's nappy rash you don't need creams, and talc is not advisable as it can be bad for their lungs. Cotton wool and water are generally considered better for a baby's skin than wipes, but if you do use wipes it's best to go for unperfumed ones, which are less likely to irritate the skin.

- If your baby is really plastered in poo, just dunk her whole bottom in a bowl of warm water – it's much more effective than dabbing away for half an hour.

THE GREAT NAPPY DEBATE

In a nutshell, the argument goes like this: disposable nappies take 200 years to biodegrade. Cloth, or 'real', nappies don't, so are probably more eco-friendly. They do need washing, but they're cheaper than disposables. Over two and a half years, you'll probably spend about £700 on nappies. The best-known types are Pampers and Huggies, but supermarket own-brand ones from Tesco and Sainsbury's are cheaper and, in my experience, just as good. The average price of branded nappies is 17.9 p per nappy. Own-brand nappies average 13.6 p per nappy. You can buy lovely eco-friendly disposables – for instance 'Nature Boy and Girl' – at Sainsbury's, Tesco and Waitrose. They are more expensive, but are seventy per cent biodegradable and very effective.

The proponents of 'real' nappies say you can buy all you need for as little as £60. See **Contacts** for more information and useful addresses.

'I remember it took Fred and me – together – over half an hour to change our first nappy,' says Sarah, mother of Hazel, twelve and Olivia, ten. 'Fortunately, it soon became significantly easier.' Midwives on wards are hideously overstretched, so you may find yourself faced with a nappy full of sticky black poo unaided. Don't panic. It's very straightforward and if you get it wrong, will the baby explode? Will she need hospital treatment? No.

Don't get paranoid about how often you change your baby's nappy – just do it whenever you notice that the nappy is dirty or wet. Initially there will be no pattern to this.

As for location, in hospital, the Perspex cot with a towel on it is a good place. In your house, a towel or changing mat on the floor is safest. Tiny babies can't officially roll, but they do wriggle, so always keep your hand on your baby if she's on a changing table to stop her falling off.

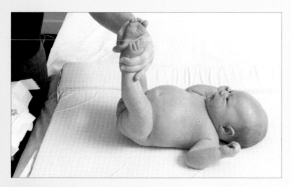

1 | Lie him on a towel and take off his dirty/ wet nappy. Use the nappy itself to scrape off any excess poo. Hold his ankles together and gently raise his bottom up a bit. Wash his bottom and genitals with cotton wool dipped in warm water. Pat him dry thoroughly with dry cotton wool (bits will stick to his bottom until it's dry) or a soft towel or muslin.

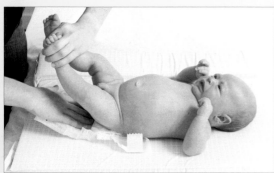

2 | When clean and dry, hold his ankles up again and slide the back half of a new nappy under his bottom.

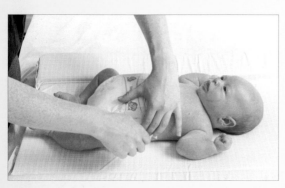

3 | Fold the top half up on to his tummy and secure it using the sticky pads from the bottom bit. Ideally, you want the sticky pads to be on his tummy, but if you put the nappy on backwards who cares? At least you've got it on. You can always get a midwife to check it when she finally comes.

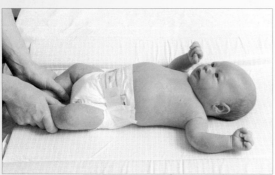

4 | Babies often poo just when you have put on a clean nappy - if it happens, just start again. Otherwise wash your hands and feel very pleased with yourself for accomplishing the first nappy change.

How to hold a newborn

Always make sure one of your hands is behind the baby's head, neck and shoulders. Most babies like to be held close to your body against your shoulder.

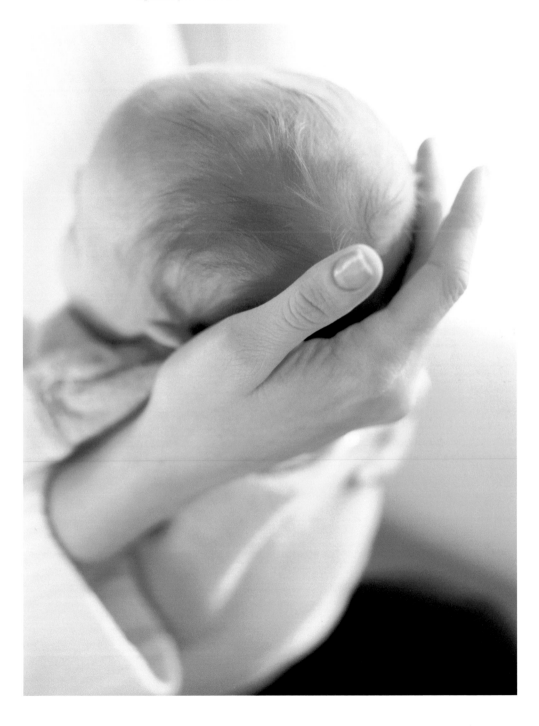

You

Your wonderful postnatal body

Or should that be 'unrecognisable'? Here are a few shockers:

- You will still look at least six months pregnant once the baby is born. It takes six weeks for your womb to shrink back to its normal size and texture.
- Your tummy will be outlandishly squishy and spongy but will gradually firm up again.
- Your stretch marks will be bright red – they'll fade to white eventually.
- Your Caesarean scar may look very raised, red and alarming – that will also fade to white eventually.

If you feel you've aged about twenty years in the last twenty-four hours, you probably have. Seriously, try not to be freaked out by all this – it's temporary and happens to us all.

How you may feel physically

You'll probably feel shockingly weak and exhausted. If you had a Caesarean it can be very difficult even to sit up. Your shoulders and legs may ache, your throat may be sore (if you spent hours baying like a beast in labour) and your eyes may be bloodshot. Luckily, you'll also have a fantastic baby – or babies – to keep your mind off it all. Indeed, you could well feel utterly elated.

If you gave birth vaginally – particularly if you tore or had an episiotomy – you're going to be seriously sore and bruised for a few days, if not weeks, and sometimes longer, though with much less intensity. Walking may be difficult and sitting down can be torture.

THERE ARE A NUMBER OF WAYS TO SOOTHE YOUR VAGINA AND PERINEUM:

- Bring a plastic jug to the hospital: pouring warm water over your bits as you pee seriously alleviates the stinging. Bring one yourself, because you'll either forget to ask the midwife or she'll be too busy to get one in time for your first pee.
- Buy 'cotton feel' maxi/maternity pads – plasticky sanitary pads can pull your stitches. Once home, keep the pads in the freezer and use them cold.

TIP

On the photos front, you may want to give your hair a brush and change out of your bloodstained birthing shirt – you're going to be looking at these photos for the rest of your life (and showing them to anything with a pulse for years).

- Dry yourself very gently: pat your vulva dry – don't rub – and don't be tempted to use the hairdryer on it because you can burn yourself.
- Consider hiring a 'valley cushion'. Available from the NCT, this is a special cushion designed to help you sit comfortably (or less agonisingly) after giving birth.
- Take any painkillers, homeopathic or herbal remedies you fancy: anything's worth a try and now is no time for stoicism.

AT HOME:

- Put bags of frozen peas in a sealed bag wrapped in a thin towel, and put them against your perineum.
- Try regular 'sitz baths' – a shallow bath in which you bathe your parts (a plastic washing-up bowl of warm water will do). Into this, herbalists at Neal's Yard Remedies recommend putting a few drops of hypericum and calendula tincture, and a few drops of lavender essential oil.

If you had a Caesarean birth, you're likely to be feeling pretty wobbly too. Here are a few ways of dealing with this.

- Again, pain relief drugs. Maximum doses. Deny yourself none.
- Get the midwife to show you alternative breastfeeding positions that don't press on your scar, which is going to be sore.
- Expect to feel weak and make sure someone is with you when you first try to get up.
- Try padding/supporting your scar by putting a sanitary towel between it and your knickers and wearing very high-waisted knickers that won't rub.
- Move: follow all the instructions you are given about movement, and get up when the midwife says you can. This will help your recovery and reduce your chances of getting a blood clot.
- Remember you just had abdominal surgery. You're bound to feel a bit dodgy.

However you gave birth, you will bleed for about seven days as if you're having an excessively heavy period; you will then have normal period-type bleeding, that gets lighter and lighter, for about a month. This is your womb shedding its lining. You might pass some freakishly large blood clots at first – tell the midwife if you pass anything larger than an ordinary-sized plum (!), if it smells foul or if you come down with a fever.

- ⊙ **Imagine you need to stop peeing halfway through: that's the muscle you're trying to use.**

- ⊙ **Clench this, tighten some more, then some more, as if going up three floors in a lift.**

- ⊙ **Hold it clenched there for about five seconds.**

- ⊙ **Then release, one 'floor' at a time.**

- ⊙ **Repeat this a few times.**

- ⊙ **Alternate this exercise with simply doing ten quick squeezes.**

- ⊙ **Try to make this a regular part of your life from now on by having daily 'triggers', such as when you go the loo, or have a drink, or get to a traffic light, or do the washing-up. You're aiming to do these exercises about ten times every day.**

As your womb starts to shrink, you'll get bad period-like cramps, known as 'afterpains', in the first twenty-four to forty-eight hours. To cope with these, use painkillers, massage your lower abdomen and lie on your stomach with a firm pillow or hot-water bottle under it if your Jordan-sized breasts allow. If you hired a TENS machine for pain relief in labour, it can help to put it back on.

There are other post-birth thrills too. Your bladder control may be practically non-existent in the first forty-eight hours or so, and decidedly dodgy for some time after. The cradle of muscles that supports your bladder and womb has been stretched by the pregnancy and birth and it needs tightening up – this will help your long-term gynaecological health, your ability to hold in pee and your sex life. Start the pelvic floor exercises along the side of this page in the first twenty-four hours. At first you may feel absolutely nothing down there, but twitch away and eventually sensation should return. If you are having any problems with this, or with incontinence, talk to your GP who can refer you to a physiotherapist. Don't be shy: this is far more common than you'd imagine.

Another delightful and common side-effect down below is piles, or haemorrhoids. These are varicose veins in your bottom that can be sore, itchy, bleed and generally make you feel like your bum has turned inside out. If you suffer from piles, don't strain to poo, get over-the-counter haemorrhoid treatments, avoid long periods of standing or sitting (lie on your side instead) and try soaking cotton wool in witch hazel and using it as a kind of soothing compress.

Constipation happens to the best of us after childbirth. It is caused by your changing hormones, but pooing a brick full of nails is the last thing you want to contend with after having a baby. So: drink tons of water – keep a jug by your bed – and get your partner to bring you fibre-rich food (hospital food is generally hopeless) like fruit (dried fruit, such as prunes, make a handy snack). When you attempt your first poo after a vaginal birth, try putting a sanitary pad over your vulva and holding firmly. This can seriously help the weird feeling that 'everything's falling out'.

Even if you've decided not to breastfeed, your boobs will produce a pale liquid called colostrum at first; after a few days they should become swollen and full of 'normal-looking' milk. If you are not breastfeeding, use breast pads and a good solid bra and your milk supply will gradually stop.

Talking of emissions – and this is the last one, honest – you'll also sweat a lot at first to expel the extra fluid your body amassed during pregnancy.

How you may feel emotionally

It's not just your body that's going to feel the after-effects of childbirth – your mind can go a bit doolally too. This is partly down to hormonal shifts, partly exhaustion and partly the sheer phenomenal experience of new parenthood. If you've just got through a particularly difficult birth, you may well feel shell-shocked by what happened. If the birth went well, you're likely to feel anything from high as a kite to completely invincible. Giving birth can genuinely make you feel you're capable of anything, and that nothing in life will ever scare or daunt you again.

Except, perhaps, keeping this wondrous infant safe and well and happy – forever. This is whopping great life stuff and it makes the early days (and weeks) of parenthood unimaginably special. But while it's going on, you're also likely, at some point, to crash. It's not surprising – birth is a big deal, both physically and emotionally, and a few nights in charge of a new and almost inconceivably precious baby, probably in a loud ward with little in the way of support, are enough to do anyone's head in. You might experience the 'baby blues' around day three, where you feel all weepy and helpless (*see page 64 for more about this*). Or you might just wobble up and down, sometimes precipitously, from time to time. All of this is normal. The best thing for you is a supportive partner who'll be there not just to hold the baby, but to hold you too sometimes. These early days of snuggling, feeding and gazing at your newborn together are what life's all about. To say it's an 'emotional time' is the understatement of the century.

The two of you: getting to know your baby

It is, of course, a massive over-simplification to say all your newborn will do is eat, sleep, excrete and cry. Your tiny being will stretch and snuffle and squeak and yawn and suck and wail and move her limbs as if she's doing an underwater dance. She'll gaze at you, or drift off to sleep, her fingers will curl and uncurl, and in her sleep her eyelids will flicker. Sometimes she'll jerk her arms and wake up shocked and howling. Sometimes she'll whimper and stir and grimace, then go back to sleep. Sometimes she'll lie so still she looks like a tiny, perfect doll and you'll wonder if she's breathing at all. I remember literally watching my baby son's eyelashes grow, hour by hour, as I fed him in the early days. For a new parent this miniature world is endlessly fascinating. It's how we get to know – and fall in love with – our babies. And it makes all the other stuff – the sleeplessness and sore bits and stitches and worries and zooming hormones – completely irrelevant. Well, some of the time, at least.

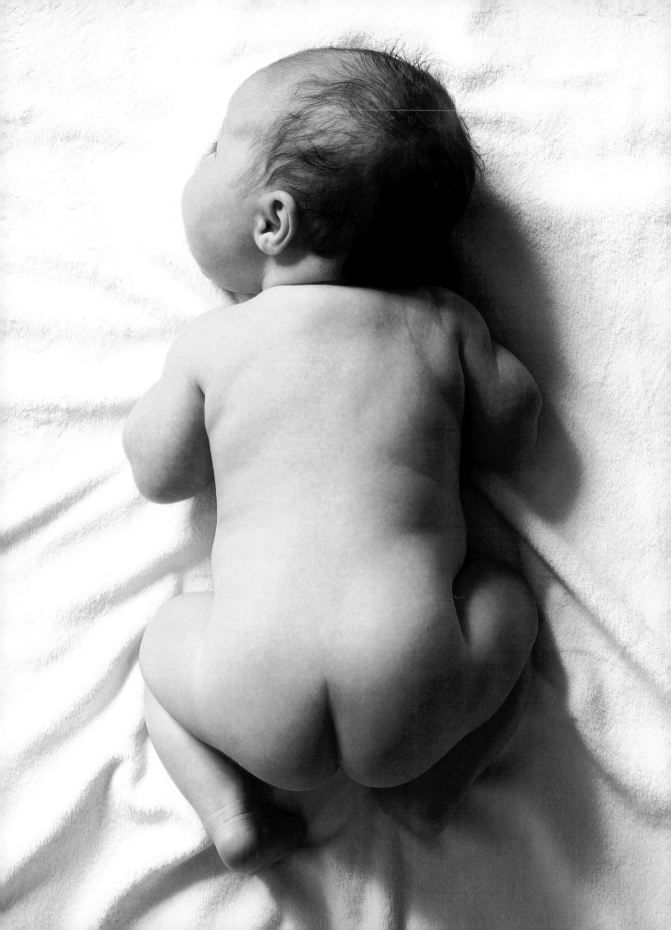

start

As you mean to go on – negotiating the first few weeks

You walk (sorry, shuffle/stagger) out into the hospital car park and it hits you: this baby, the one you're carrying now in his teeny car seat, in the outside world, is *yours*. It's an amazing feeling. It's also slightly terrifying. How can they expect you to look after him completely unaided? It's the new-parent wake-up call and it happens to us all: life will – truly – never be the same again.

THESE ARE THE TOP TEN NEW-PARENT WORRIES:

1 | Will my baby die? (Yes, we all worry about it.)
2 | Is my baby healthy and normal?
3 | Am I doing it right?
4 | Is my baby eating enough/too much/at the right times?
5 | Is my baby crying too much?
6 | Is my baby sleeping too much/too little/at the wrong times?
7 | Will I ever feel like 'myself' again?
8 | Will my relationship ever recover?
9 | How are we going to afford this?
10 | Will I be a good parent?

This chapter is your basic guide to getting through – and hopefully enjoying – the first few weeks. This includes, of course, coping superlatively with all of the above worries.

Getting your baby home

THERE ARE CERTAIN THINGS YOUR BABY WILL NEED FOR HIS DEPARTURE FROM HOSPITAL.

- A car seat *suitable from birth (see page 21)*
- Clothes: vest, Babygro, socks, cotton hat and cardigan (unless it's hot)
- A warm outer garment if it's winter
- A cellular or lightweight blanket if it's summer, unless it's hot. Use your common sense or, if this has deserted you, ask a midwife.

AND YOU WILL NEED:

- Drugs. Take whatever pain meds you can get, at least forty-five minutes before you have to 'walk' to your car.
- Clothes. No, no, the Diesel jeans won't work – this season you'll mostly be wearing elasticated waistbands in very large sizes.
- Nerves of steel.

A good tip is to stuff your baby with milk and burp him well *(see page 54 for how)* just before you leave. That way you can rule out hunger when he starts to yell (which he almost certainly will). Though your baby looks tiny, he's relatively robust for someone that small. You're in this together and if you want to enjoy the next few months you have – to a certain extent – to force yourself not to sweat the small stuff. From now, and for the foreseeable future, this is a very valuable thing to remind yourself of.

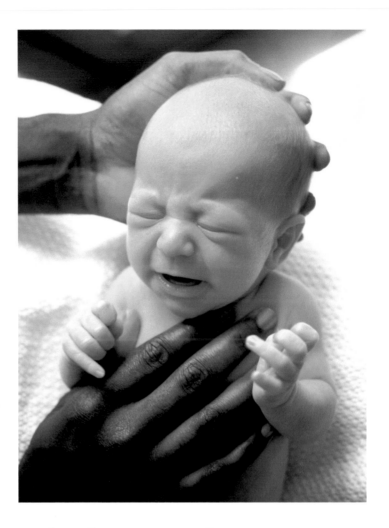

What to do when you get home

'The whole world feels fragile now, as if I were carrying my heart around,' says Melissa, mother of Raphael, nine months. If this throws you into a tizzy for the first few weeks, you're not alone. 'I felt total panic at home with my new baby,' says Julia, mother of Charlie, one. 'He seemed so fragile and the sense of responsibility was just overwhelming. Instead of gazing at my baby in this bubble of maternal love, I just kept thinking, He's so important, what if something happened to him?'

Not everyone feels worried. But if you do, the anxiety should subside once you get to know your baby a bit and gain confidence. If it doesn't, it's important to talk to your midwife or health visitor about how you feel (excessive anxiety, apart from being distracting, can be a sign of postnatal depression).

The main thing is to get to know your baby. 'He didn't come with any instructions and I couldn't speak his language,' says Lori, mother of Jacob, two. 'I felt like I was failing all the time.' Be kind to yourself here. You will slowly learn – your way – that he won't break if you put his nappy on wrong, or explode if you take too long to do his poppers up (though he may shout a lot). He doesn't have some pre-programmed need to be held or spoken to in the 'right' way, and he doesn't know any better than you do how he should be bathed or fed. The right way, in short, is *your* fumbling, inept, loving and slowly evolving way.

FIVE TOP TIPS FOR THE FIRST FEW WEEKS:

1 | Take a babymoon *(see below)*.
2 | Get help *(see below)*. Lots of it.
3 | Shelve all normal tasks: tidying, bill-paying and sending out birth announcements can all wait.
4 | Sleep whenever you get the chance (even a half-hour catnap is better than nothing).
5 | Only have visitors on your terms: ask people to leave, cancel their visits, only let them stay a very short time – normal sociability rules do not apply.

A word about visitors

Remember, it's *your* baby and you are allowed to do things *your* way – no matter who you offend. Josie, mother of Kofi, fifteen weeks, remembers that her biggest difficulty during the early weeks was with visitors. 'I often felt that they did not appreciate my need to be with my baby. With hindsight I should have been more assertive. I found it very hard to watch people pass Kofi from one person to another when I just wanted to hold and protect him.'

THE PAPARAZZI
There's one thing most of us worry about that we needn't: flash photography by the granny paparazzi is not going to hurt your baby's eyes, induce epileptic fits or damage anything other than your sanity.

A babymoon

Your priority as a new mother should not be to slim yourself concave in the first four weeks. Your body and mind need to adjust and recover. A significantly better way to embark on motherhood is to have a 'babymoon'. Just snuggle up with your baby and do little else but eat, sleep and feed for a good week after the birth.

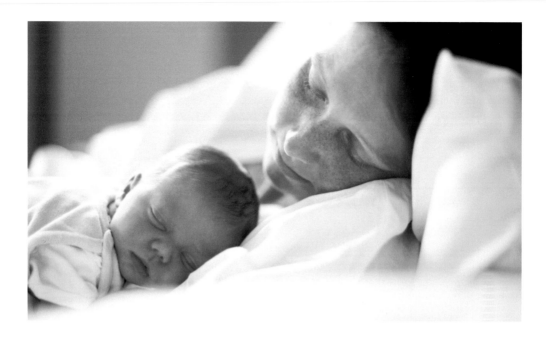

TO HAVE THE IDEAL BABYMOON:

- Stay in your pyjamas for at least three days.
- Have lots of skin-to-skin contact with your baby (this is a great thing for dads to do too, but is particularly important for the mother if she is breastfeeding).
- Eat meals you have cooked and frozen already. You want things that can be reheated quickly and don't require accompaniments – one-pot meals such as soups and stews that include veggies. They should preferably be heated up (and cleared away) by someone else.
- Stay in bed a lot. Have all the things you need to change your baby's nappy and clothes in one place. Have a large bottle of water and some snacks nearby. Just chill out together.

Help!

You will need to establish who, while you are chilling out with your newborn in the first couple of weeks, will prepare and clear up the meals, do the shopping, clean the house and do the laundry (there will be lots of it). It's a mistake to assume that the dad will be the one to do all of this. As a dad, your role will inevitably include a bit of popping out to the shop, tidying up, making cups of tea or sticking the odd load of laundry on;

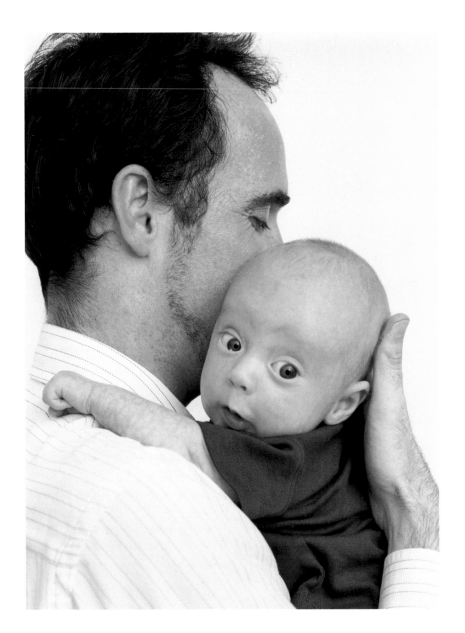

but it's a good idea to get some other help too, so you can snuggle with your partner and baby and enjoy this time together. The baby needs to bond with his father too (and vice versa).

If you can, try and set up help in advance for cooking, cleaning, shopping and basic household tasks, and accept whatever else you can get. 'Being able to accept help is so important,' says Julia. 'My mum offered to help burp and settle him in the night, but I said, "No, I have to learn, I'm his mother." In retrospect this was a bit silly. You should take all the help you can get, when you can get it.'

Your help options *(starting with the poshest)*

MATERNITY NURSE

She lives in and usually comes for the first week or two to help you all adjust. **Cost:** about £600 a week, via an agency. To find one try www.nannydirectory.co.uk or nanny agencies in your area.

NIGHT NANNY

She'll stay in your house from about 9 p.m.–7 a.m. If you are breastfeeding she will bring the baby to your room for feeds and take him away afterwards, doing all the jiggling and nappy-changing while you recuperate. **Cost:** around £70 per night. To find one try www.all4kidsuk.com or ring around your local nanny agencies.

POSTNATAL DOULA

She's like a very experienced best friend (only you don't feel guilty) who comes for a few hours a day to help you bond with your baby and rest. She'll advise on anything from feeding to equipment, and will help with things like shopping and light housework. Not available in all parts of the country (yet). **Cost:** £10–£15 per hour. To find one try Doula UK, www.doula.org.uk.

MOTHERS' HELPS

Basically, you pay a sensible local teenage girl to help you around the house – washing-up, laundry, hoovering, jiggling the baby's pram, changing the odd nappy, answering the front door. Be clear, in advance, exactly what her duties will be. Expect her to be fickle (i.e. she may not show up), and don't ask her to look after your baby for longer than about half an hour unattended. **Cost:** £4–£5 per hour, or whatever you can get away with. To find one try friends, neighbours or your local community college (they often have childcare diplomas, and some students may be looking for work).

FAMILY AND FRIENDS

Mums, if you are lucky enough to have one who can come, tend to be heaven in the weeks after their grandchild's arrival. But be clear about what you want your family members to do. Cook? Clear up? Take the baby for walks? The golden rule is if they're stressing you out, get them to leave (tell them that they've been great, but you realise you need to get used to the baby on your own – or something like that). And have a back-up plan. **Cost:** only you can know the answer to this one.

The professionals

Getting advice generally isn't the problem – everyone from the granny in Tesco to the builder and his mate will share their baby tips with you. A far greater challenge is sorting the good advice from the rubbish advice. If in doubt, trust your instincts. 'After a few weeks I stopped being so paranoid,' says Ginny, mother of Phoebe, nine months. 'I realised that no one had ever been my daughter's mother before so I shouldn't judge myself on other people's criteria.'

However, if you understand what people are there for, the NHS postnatal support network can get you a long way.

The midwife

TO GET THE BEST FROM YOUR MIDWIFE'S VISITS:

⊙ **Talk to her specifically about anything that's worrying you and get answers. Write things down so you remember them.**

⊙ **Get information about who to call night or day if something is worrying you, and put the numbers somewhere obvious like your fridge door.**

⊙ **Don't be afraid to cry or take up her time.**

⊙ **Don't think you have to tidy up. She's seen far worse.**

⊙ **If you are feeling desperate, anxious or like you're not coping, tell her clearly how you feel.**

In most parts of the UK, a midwife will visit you at home regularly for about a week to make sure you're recovering from the birth and to check that your baby is healthy and eating well.

When your baby is six to twelve days old, the midwife or health visitor *(see below)* will do a heel-prick test on him. She pricks your baby's heel and collects a few droplets of blood to screen for certain developmental conditions including a thyroid deficiency called hypothyroidism and a rare condition called phenylketonuria (PKU). If you feed your baby while the heel prick happens, he'll notice it less. You in your hormonal state, may well burst into tears at this point. Your baby will be fine.

Health visitors

Usually – in most parts of the UK – between the tenth and the fourteenth day after you have your baby you'll start getting a weekly visit from your health visitor. These will last for about six weeks. Health visitors are nurses or midwives with special training in child health and health promotion. Their job is to check your baby's development and growth, and make sure you are coping with parenthood. If you don't hear from a health visitor in the first couple of weeks, tell your midwife or GP.

YOUR HEALTH VISITOR WILL DO THE FOLLOWING:

● Bring a Personal Child Health Record booklet for you to keep and bring to any visits to the baby clinic, doctor or hospital appointments. This is your record of your baby's growth, check-ups and immunisations.
● Weigh (and sometimes measure) your baby

- Ask how he is feeding, and give advice if necessary
- Ask how you are doing physically
- Check how you and your partner are coping generally
- Tell you about immunisations, future check-ups and postnatal depression
- Ask about your life in general in terms of housing and family health
- Help you come up with a plan for getting any further support if necessary

Baby clinics

After the initial period of home visits, you'll be asked to bring your baby along to see the health visitor for regular weigh-ins, check-ups and immunisations. Most health visitors run weekly baby clinics, usually at the GP's surgery. If anything is worrying you between baby clinics, call the health visitor. It's fine to turn up at the baby clinic even if your baby isn't 'due' a check-up – it's a good place to go to get advice and talk through any worries. But you certainly don't *have* to go every week.

Your six-week check

This is normally done by your GP, who needs to check that your body has recovered properly from pregnancy and childbirth. Your doctor will check that your bleeding has stopped and any stitches have healed. She'll check your heart and blood pressure, will ask you about contraception, and should check when you last had a cervical smear test.

Newborn peculiarities

Newborns can be perplexing: strange blisters, bumps and rashes pop up with alarming regularity. Here are some of the first worries you may encounter.

Skin

RASHES

Little yellow or white pinhead spots on the face are 'milia' or 'baby acne'. They are caused by inexperienced skin glands unplugging themselves and are very common in the first few days and weeks.

They are totally harmless. Tiny, flat, red pinhead spots, mostly on the face, neck and torso, may be heat rash. If your baby seems happy and healthy, rashes are usually not something to worry about; but if in doubt, always ask your health visitor. If your baby seems unwell (for example has a fever) with any rash, or if a rash seems to be getting worse, see your GP. Some serious illnesses like meningitis may come with a rash, but your baby will be obviously very unwell if this is happening – *see page 165.*

Mouth

SUCKING BLISTERS

White blisters on the lips are common, don't need treatment and should disappear in the first few weeks.

THRUSH

This is a common yeast infection of the baby's mouth: it looks as if patches of milk curd are stuck to your baby's cheeks, tongue or the roof of his mouth (they won't wipe off). This does need medicine so see your GP for a prescription.

Eyes

STICKY EYES

One or both eyes ooze or stick together when your baby has been asleep. This is usually just an irritation from the fluids your baby has encountered at birth. To treat it, wipe your baby's eyes with cooled boiled water (use a different piece of cotton wool for each eye) from the inner corner then outwards, every few hours.

BLOCKED TEAR DUCT

This is also common – white gooey stuff collects in the corner and edges of the eyelids, which can get stuck together. The eye may also seem 'weepy'. Treat as for sticky eyes, and massage your baby's tear duct several times a day by gently rubbing it at the side of the nose, beneath the corner of the eye. If regular cleaning and massaging for a day or so is not helping, or anything seems to be getting worse (with this or sticky eyes), see your GP – it could be conjunctivitis, an infection that is contagious and often treated with antibiotic eye drops.

CROSSED OR SQUINTY EYES

These are common in the first twelve weeks or so because a baby's eyes don't work together yet. Talk to your GP if the squinting goes on beyond three months.

Scalp

Some new babies get a swelling on the scalp because of bleeding under the skin at birth. This is normal, won't do any harm, and can take a few weeks to go away (show your health visitor if you are anxious). Most babies also get cradle cap – scaly, flaky skin on the scalp. It's not dandruff or scurvy, and you can remove some of it by massaging the top of your baby's head with olive oil. Or just ignore it – it's normal and harmless and will go away eventually.

The umbilical cord stump

The stump will drop off somewhere between five and ten days. It's best just to leave it alone and be gentle when bathing/dressing your baby (it's fine to get it wet, but pat it dry carefully). A bulging navel, however, might indicate an 'umbilical hernia', so if you notice this, call your GP or health visitor: these are usually harmless but can take up to a year to go away. If you notice that the stump is oozing pus or discharge, is very stinky or looks red, call the midwife or your GP the same day as it could be infected.

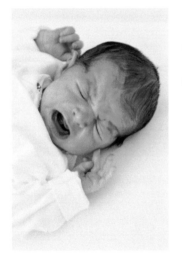

See **Chapter Five** for the low-down on crying.

Chapter Six will give you the feeding basics from day one to one year.

Some things your baby will do

Cry

If your baby was all peaceful and sleepy for the first few days then goes off like a siren on day three, you may or may not find small comfort in the knowledge that this is entirely normal. It often coincides with your return from hospital and the shock of being *alone* and – supposedly – *in charge*, and it can shake your confidence. It also tends to coincide with the dad's return to work, so it's no wonder many new mothers feel they're not a 'natural'. At least some of the time, you are bound to feel despairing, worried, angry or desperate about your baby's cries. You wouldn't be a parent if you didn't.

Eat

By now you've decided how you'll be feeding your baby. Or have you? For some new parents, feeding the baby is totally straightforward. For the rest of us it is, initially, a changeable scenario. It may take a few weeks to establish feeding properly, and you may need help and support, particularly if you are breastfeeding.

There are also some by-products of your baby's eating, and you should know how to deal with them.

WIND

A baby that's taking in too much air with his milk will writhe around, tuck his legs up towards his chest and probably cry after or during a feed. He may make loud sucking noises at the bottle or breast. 'Trapped wind is the number-one problem I see with parents and newborns,' says baby consultant Su Moulana. 'You have to learn to wind your baby properly, so that he can get enough milk at every feed and settle well afterwards.'

There is probably no harm in trying products like gripe water and Infacol that help babies burp up trapped wind (you can buy them in chemists and some supermarkets). I had three very windy babies and tried all sorts of things. Eventually with Ted, my third, I went to a breastfeeding specialist who showed me how to latch him on properly. He turned from a writhing windy baby to a calm, peaceful one overnight – something gallons of gripe water had not achieved.

Good wind-minimising strategies depend on whether you are bottle-feeding or breastfeeding.

IF YOU ARE BOTTLE-FEEDING:

- Check that when you're tilting the bottle, the teat and neck are filled with milk (there should be no visible air).
- Try sitting him in a more upright position as you feed him.
- Try switching to a different brand of feeding bottle or formula (ask your health visitor for advice on appropriate brands).

IF YOU ARE BREASTFEEDING:

- Get help with your latch-on technique. It is the number-one cause of windy babies.
- Some people say breastfed babies can react windily to certain foods in your diet: the main culprits are cruciferous vegetables like broccoli, and obvious things that make *you* windy, like beans and cabbage.

However, this is not true according to UNICEF breastfeeding experts. While tastes are transmitted in breast milk, gas is not, and nor is fibre (which makes *you* windy). If your baby is unsettled, it is far more likely to be your latch-on than your diet.

FARTING

They can be as loud as an adult's and still entirely normal. If, however, they are accompanied by a lot of crying and writhing, your baby may be getting too much air with his feeds.

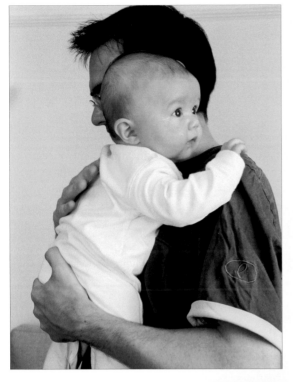

SO HOW DO YOU BURP YOUR BABY?

1 | Lay him against your shoulder.

2 | Straighten his body and legs out by stroking down his back and legs firmly. You want his belly flat against you.

3 | Gently pat or rub his back rhythmically until a burp comes out.

4 | You can also wind your baby by sitting him on your lap, supporting his head and chest under his chin while you rub or pat his back with your other hand. Keep his back straight.

5 | If nothing comes out after about thirty seconds there may be nothing there, but you have to get to know your own baby on this one.

6 | Try this mid-feed if he seems uncomfortable or is pulling away but hasn't had much milk.

THROWING UP

Often called, delicately, 'possetting' or 'spitting up', your baby's sick can be quite frequent and copious and yet still normal. Be aware, however, that if he throws up a lot after a feed he may be hungrier sooner than a baby who holds it all down.

HERE ARE THREE SICK-MINIMISING THINGS TO TRY:

1 | Burp him halfway through a feed and avoid bouncing him around too much afterwards.
2 | If bottle-feeding, check that the teat is suitable for his age. They come in different 'flow' sizes: slow for newborns, getting faster for bigger babies. If the flow is too fast, it may cause him to throw up. You can also ask your health visitor about other feeding-bottle teats that might help.
3 | If breastfeeding, check that he is latched on well.

TALK TO YOUR GP IF:

- He's not just bringing up what's just been drunk but is vomiting more copiously, or the sick looks different than usual – not just like curdling milk. Brown or green or very projectile vomiting should also be checked out by a doctor.
- He is throwing up frequently and not gaining weight.
- He is gagging or coughing a lot.
- He seems to be in pain.
- You're just worried.

'Don't call social services on yourself if you open your baby's nappy to find a Belisha beacon glaring back at you. But do take measures to soothe it.'

REFLUX

This is caused by stomach acid and milk flowing back up the throat during and after feeds. Your baby will be obviously distressed or 'colicky' (i.e. in pain, yelling, inconsolable) usually after or during a feed. Talk to your doctor if this seems to be happening.

HICCUPING

Perfectly normal and common in new babies, hiccups don't bother the baby as much as they would you, and usually abate as he gets bigger.

Poo

Your baby's poos should be soft, watery and generally a light brown or mustardy yellow colour, though don't worry if they are sometimes green. Thankfully, few parents are actively revolted by their own baby's poo (although someone else's baby is a whole different ball game). Almost all babies sometimes do explosive poos, taking out an entire outfit, usually in public when you've forgotten your nappy bag. This does not mean they're ill or even uncomfortable.

Pooing after every feed or more is perfectly normal in the early weeks (the floodgates should close as your baby gets older). It is also normal – especially for breastfed babies – to poo as little as once every three or four days, or even once a week.

You should talk to your doctor if the poos are very frequent, watery and bad-smelling, if they have mucus in them, and if they are accompanied by a fever – it could be diarrhoea *(see page 164)*. You should also talk to the doctor if the poos are hard, pellet-like and obviously cause him pain, or even bleeding as they come out. He could be constipated, although a bit of straining or brief discomfort is normal.

Change his nappy whenever he seems wet, and definitely whenever he poos. In the first few weeks this may happen ten or twelve times a day. It helps to have a 'nappy station' somewhere (ideally next to a sink) with your cotton wool, clean Babygros, towels and muslins all in one place.

If your baby's bottom gets red and raw-looking, it could be nappy rash, usually caused by prolonged contact with pee or poo. Almost all babies get it at some point (girls seem to get it more easily than boys). Strong soaps or bubble baths can also cause nappy rash, as can wipes containing alcohol, and a period of illness. In other words, don't call social services on yourself if you open your baby's nappy to find a Belisha beacon glaring back at you. But do take measures to soothe it:

- Wash and dry the area thoroughly.
- Lie your baby on a towel and let him be nappy-free for as long and as often as you can.
- Slather a barrier cream on the red bits once your baby is clean and dry, before putting the nappy back on. Sudocrem is a well-known brand available in chemists or supermarkets; Neal's Yard does a good 'natural' alternative (www.nealsyardremedies.com).
- You don't need to use a barrier cream once your baby's bottom has healed: it's generally better for the skin to breathe.

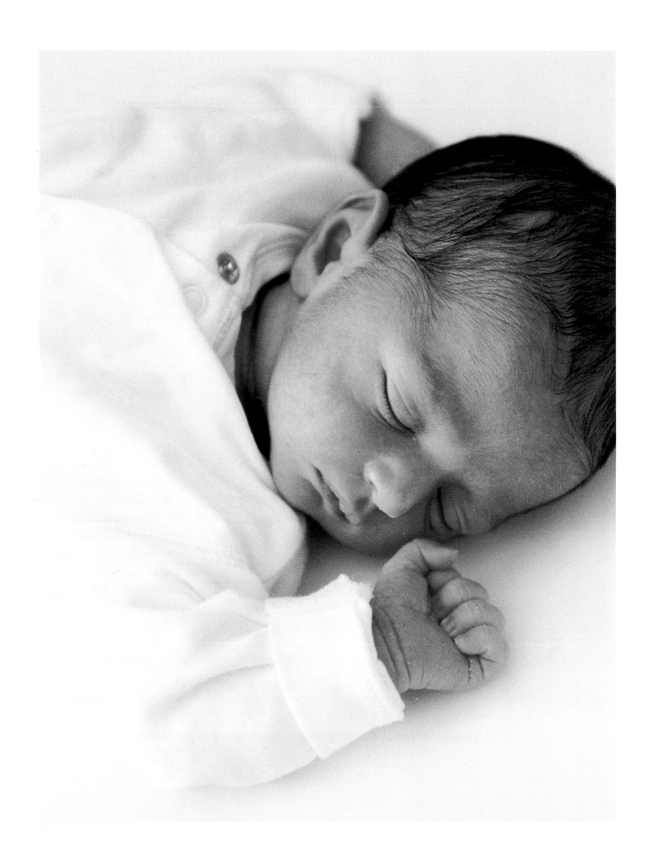

Sleep

New babies don't know the difference between night and day, and they need to eat every couple of hours, so sleep deprivation is a *huge* part of any new parent's life. In the first two or three weeks it is not worth getting obsessed about routines and schedules. Your baby will need lots of cuddles and feeds and will probably have no discernable sleep routines. But bear in mind, as your first few weeks pass, that in the long term a laissez-faire approach may not be your best bet.

For ways to help your baby become a prize sleeper, see **Chapter Four**.

Basic Skills

Baby handling

As long as you are supporting his head and neck there's no right way to hold and lift your baby – just work out what feels right to you both.

After the first couple of weeks he'll probably start to like lying on a mat or rug, kicking and wriggling, with you nearby. Think of this as baby aerobics. And don't forget to put him on his tummy sometimes to kick around: this strengthens the neck and back and might help him expel some wind – from either end – too.

When he's a few weeks old you can start to put him in a sling-type bouncy seat on the floor – not the table – where he can watch you cook or bustle around the room. The car seat isn't a good place for a baby to sit for long periods as it doesn't give good back support.

Most new babies object violently to being dressed, so expect a lot of stressful fumbling at first. The top tips are: lie him somewhere soft and warm, stretch the necks of vests and T-shirts before you pull them over his head, keep a hand on his belly for reassurance when he's naked, and pop up the poppers from the top to bottom as that way you're less likely to do it all wrong and have to start again.

Don't be afraid to let other people cuddle your baby. One popular childcare book says that if someone touches your newborn, you should surreptitiously pull out a wipe to remove the germs from your baby's skin. Unless your baby is very premature or sick, this is the behaviour of a lunatic. Other people touching your baby will do him *no harm whatsoever*. Of course, if the person touching him has some appallingly contagious condition, or is a dangerous madman, think again. But generally, people who just love babies will do yours no harm.

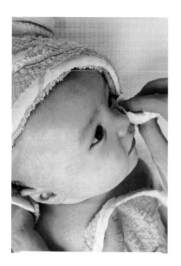

Keeping your baby clean

A bath a couple of times a week, or whenever he's got poo or sick all over him, is all you need, but a daily wash of hands, face and bottom ('topping and tailing') is a good idea. Ideally do this when he is rested, fed and happy (i.e. that brief two-minute slot in your otherwise lunatic day).

To do this you'll need a warm room, a bowl or sink of warm water, a bowl of cooled boiled water, a towel, a roll of cotton wool and a fresh nappy. Hold him (dressed) on your knee or lie him on his changing mat and wipe the outside of his ears (not the inside), the folds of his neck and his hands. Wipe his eyes with cotton wool dipped in cooled boiled water (a different piece for each eye – you boil then cool the eye-washing water to avoid infections). Pat everything dry, then change his nappy.

HOW TO BATH YOUR BABY

There is really no science to bathing a baby: you just have to keep him basically clean without drowning him.

YOU'LL NEED:

- A receptacle: a washing-up bowl, a sink, your normal bath or a special baby bath, which your baby will outgrow within a few months. (Put any receptacle on the floor or inside your bath so it can't fall off a surface.)
- A towel (oh, go on, make it soft and warm ...)
- A clean nappy
- Clean clothes
- A roll of cotton wool
- Mild baby wash as your baby gets bigger and smellier
- A warm bathroom
- You might find a bath thermometer reassuring.

A word about baby 'products': paediatric dermatologists (baby-skin specialists) have expressed concerns that the rise in asthma, eczema and allergies is linked in part to the burgeoning market in baby soaps, shampoos, bubble baths and lotions. As your baby gets bigger and smellier, you will need mild shampoo or baby wash, but I'd use the minimum number of products you need to keep your baby's skin and hair basically clean and comfortable. Until he's about eight weeks old, you really just need warm water. I tend to go for products made with as few chemicals as possible, but that's just me. Green People do a good baby wash developed by the mother of a child with severe

A FEW TIPS:

- Use a different piece of cotton wool for bum/each eye/mouth so you don't transfer germs.

- Never poke cotton wool into ears, nose or any orifice.

- Don't pull the foreskin back or clean inside the labia – they are, handily, 'self-cleaning' and you can actually do harm by trying to clean them.

- For the first ten days or so just clean around the umbilical stump. It is fine for it to get wet in the bath – just pat it dry afterwards.

eczema (www.greenpeople.co.uk). Green Baby is also a good organic brand (www.greenbaby.co.uk). If your baby does develop eczema or any other skin complaint, you should get specialist advice on products and treatments *(see page 165)*.

To bath your baby, slip one arm under his neck and shoulders and hold under his armpit so he won't slip under the water. Scoop water over him with your free hand, then pat him gently dry, making sure you dab into the creases and under his arms and chin. To wash his hair (once or twice a week is fine) lean him back, scoop some water over his head and wash using a mild shampoo or baby wash.

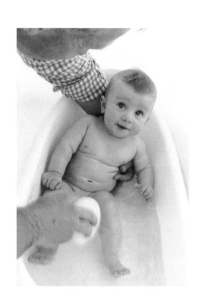

Some babies hate bath time and are hysterical throughout; others think it's heaven. Having a bath together can be reassuring for babies that don't like being naked or bathed alone (use non-slip mats so you don't fall while holding him). One friend of mine revolutionised her six-month-old son's bath time simply by showing him the bath while she put him in, rather than undressing him and plonking him in backwards. After all, you'd probably shout, too, if you were suddenly and unexpectedly submerged in tepid water.

TWO GOLDEN SAFETY RULES

1 | Check the water is not too hot: your baby's skin is thinner and more sensitive than yours and will scald very, very easily. The water should be at roughly your body temperature. Put your elbow in to test it (your hand may not be as temperature-sensitive).

2 | Never leave your baby alone in the bath: drowning is one of the most common causes of death in babies and young children, who can drown in an inch of water. Never *ever* leave your baby alone in the bath, even for a second to answer a phone, rush out for a nappy or whatever, even when he can sit up alone.

'Some babies hate bath time and are hysterical throughout; others think it's heaven.'

DON'T PANIC, CAPTAIN MAINWARING!

Most of us have, at some point, accidentally let the baby slip under the water. As long as you fish him up again *instantly* – which will be your overriding instinct anyway – you don't need to turn yourself in to the police. It's shocking when it happens and he may yell pitifully afterwards, but a moment's unexpected dip is not going to do him any harm.

NAILS

The easiest way to keep your baby's nails short is by biting them off yourself. Alternatively, use special blunt baby-nail scissors. Scratch mitts are a bit of a shame: a baby really needs to be discovering the world with his fingers.

The outside world

When you first go out with your baby, you might feel like the world is watching you, poised to pounce on your every mistake. It is not. Many of the grown-ups you'll meet are parents and are therefore on your side. The rest are not remotely interested, and think babies cry all the time anyway. A short walk, with your baby in the sling or buggy, is a good first outing. Try to go with your partner, mum or best friend for moral support. And expect yelling – your baby is not used to noise, bright lights and funny smells, or the feel of a buggy.

WHAT NOT TO WEAR

The basic rule is that your baby should wear roughly the amount of clothing you'd feel comfortable in yourself, but he will get hot or cold quite a lot quicker than you would if the temperature changes.

You

Your crazy body

It may feel alien but bear with it: it's done a spectacular thing.

Your womb won't shrink back to its former size for at least six weeks, your periods may not return for six months or so, you're unlikely to lose all your baby fat for at least nine months (and often much longer) and you may, for a while, feel achy in your pelvis and back from the strains of pregnancy.

TO RECOVER WELL, YOUR BODY NEEDS:

- Rest when humanly possible
- Regular, nutritious meals whenever you can manage this
- Some gentle exercise
- Your patience and undying gratitude

Here are a few guidelines to help you do some gentle but effective exercise.

A FEW BABY TEMPERATURE TIPS:

- Take off hats, coats, blankets or extra clothes as soon as you come into a warm building, even if your baby is asleep.

- Feel his tummy or back to check how hot or cold he is as his hands and feet will be generally colder than yours anyway.

- Keep him in a cotton hat unless it's very warm, as he'll lose a lot of heat from his head.

- Keep him in cotton (not synthetic) clothes in hotter weather as they let the skin breathe.

- Take an extra blanket in case it gets chilly.

- Keep babies under six months out of the sun entirely. Always put a sun hat on him, and use sunscreen (SPF15) for babies over six months.

DAY ONE TO AT LEAST SIX WEEKS AFTER GIVING BIRTH

Your body still contains the hormone relaxin after the birth. This makes your ligaments more liable to strain, so don't even think about doing aerobic or strenuous exercise until your doctor says it's OK (usually at your six-week check-up, though up to three months if you had a Caesarean).

IN THE MEANTIME, DO THESE EXERCISES A FEW TIMES A DAY:

- Pelvic floor exercises *(see page 40)*
- Abdominal tightenings: slowly breathe in, pushing your belly outwards to the count of five, then breathe out slowly, pulling your belly back towards your spine again. Repeat ten times.
- Head lifts: lie on your back with your arms at your sides, knees bent, feet placed hip width apart on the floor. Inhale, raise your head slightly, exhaling as you do. Lower it back, inhaling slowly. Do this about ten times.
- Leg slides: using the same position as above, slide your right foot towards your bum, then slowly lift your right knee towards your chest. Slide back down. Repeat with the other leg. Do this about five times with each leg.
- Short, gentle strolls: once you're up to it, try going for short strolls (about twenty minutes to start with) with your baby in a sling or buggy.

Your health visitor should give you detailed information about other safe postnatal exercises, and you may want to sign up to your hospital's postnatal exercise class (usually to begin after your six-week check).

AFTER SIX WEEKS

Once exercise has been OK'd by your doctor, you should be able to pick up your exercising life where you left off (though you'll be considerably less fit). If you previously did nothing but sit on the sofa and now want overall healthy living, walking briskly for half an hour five times a week with your baby in the stroller is all it takes. If you want to get fitter (and maybe lose some baby weight) you're going to have to raise your heart rate for about thirty to forty minutes at least three or four times a week, doing something mildly strenuous like jogging, an exercise class or vigorous swimming. Experts say the key to success is to reserve a set time for exercise when you know you have someone to look after your baby, and ideally exercise with a 'buddy'. Many gyms and leisure centres now have crèche facilities.

Postnatal depression and the baby blues

Sometimes parenthood is just a straightforward downer. 'I had to accept my own scary temptation to launch him/myself out the window sometimes,' says Madeline, mother of Tola, nine months. Mothers don't tend to admit the really bad bits (on some level I suspect we're scared people will think we don't love our babies if we express the dark side). But we all, occasionally, think these grim things.

On or around days three to five after the birth, about fifty per cent of new mothers feel weepy, depressed, desperate or helpless. Known as the 'baby blues', this is a normal mood response to precipitous drops in your hormones in the first few days after giving birth (combined with exhaustion and heightened emotions). The baby blues can go on for up to fourteen days, but usually they just last a day or two if that.

'I went from being ecstatically happy and bursting with pride … to pulling my hair out.'

Ten to fifteen per cent of new mothers develop postnatal depression (PND) – a completely separate condition to baby blues. It is way more than just a couple of days feeling weepy, and can start, slowly or suddenly, at any point in the first year. It is a treatable illness, but it is often missed by partners, family, friends and health professionals, sometimes with catastrophic consequences (one to two per cent of new mothers develop a severe illness called postnatal psychosis).

You and, crucially, your partner should keep an eye out for the warning signs of PND. You may have symptoms similar to the baby blues, *and* you may have any combination of these symptoms:

- Despondency and hopelessness
- Feeling exhausted all the time
- Being unable to concentrate
- Feeling guilt/inadequacy
- Anxiety, feeling unable to cope
- Feeling uninterested in the baby
- Feeling hyper-concerned about the baby
- Obsessive thoughts
- Panic
- Fear of harming yourself or your baby

- Headaches/chest pains
- Not caring about your appearance
- Sleeplessness (even when the baby is not waking you)
- Losing your appetite

The warning signs of severe PND or postnatal psychosis include the above symptoms, but you may also:

- Seem confused
- Have severe mood swings
- Feel hopeless or ashamed
- Talk about suicide/hurting the baby
- Seem hyperactive or manic
- Talk quickly or incoherently
- Act suspiciously or seem fearful of everything
- Have delusions or hallucinations

The medication used for PND may be different to that used for general kinds of depression, so if your depression isn't acknowledged as PND, you can go on suffering for ages on the wrong treatment. If you think you (or someone you know) may have PND, treatment from a specialist is essential. See **Contacts** for organisations and books that may help.

Ultimately, once you get through the panicky early days, can change nappies, jiggle, feed and generally cope most of the time, the good bits about parenthood tend to outweigh the bad bits a thousand-fold. Here's what a few new parents say:

'I've been surprised by how overwhelmed you are with love for your baby'
'My baby has made me a better person'
'I look forward to every day and feel complete in a way I didn't before'

Parenthood is, clearly, one of life's big uppers. It can be a rollercoaster too: 'I went from being ecstatically happy and bursting with pride, thinking I had mastered the knack pretty quickly and had it sussed,' says Laura, mother of Reuben, four months, 'to pulling my hair out knowing that nothing I did made any difference to this screaming baby and wondering why oh why had I wanted to have a baby.'

Your baby's first smile can, however, genuinely dwarf the wailing and sleeplessness and chaos that went before. As one mother I interviewed for this book put it, 'I'm surprised at how amazing being a parent is. However bad the day is, I look at James smile and my heart melts.'

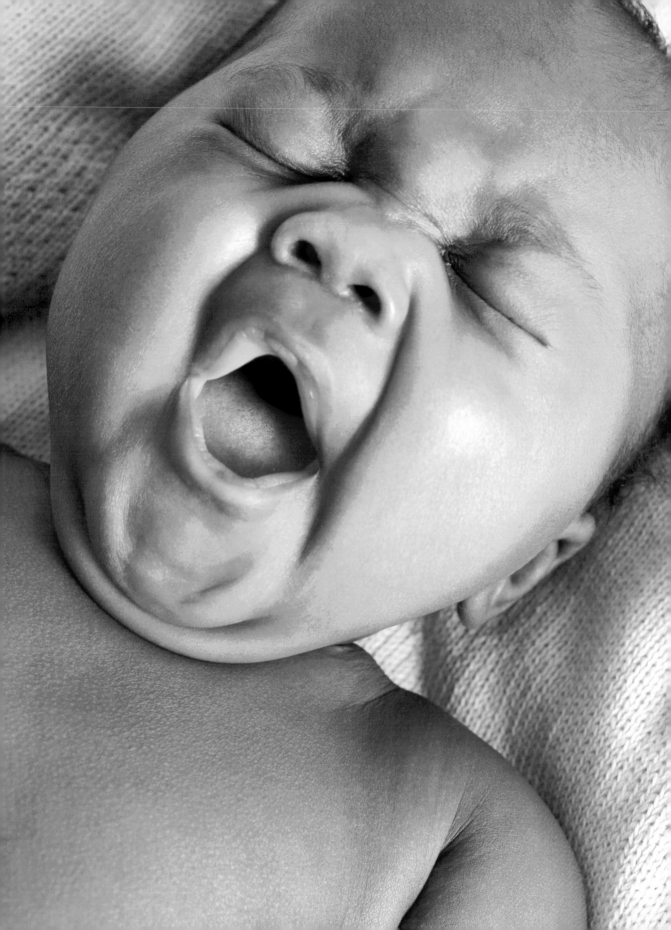

sleep

How to get some (all of you)

Hormones, adrenaline and sheer new-baby delight can get you a long way at first. But sleep deprivation, if it goes on for a while (and it probably will) can become tough. It's a form of torture, after all. Coping strategies are essential if you're not to go stark staring mad. It's also a sensible idea to do things, from very early on, to encourage your baby to become a prize sleeper (i.e. not wake you up seven times a night until she's a preschooler). So here's the lowdown on sleep: how much your baby needs, why she'll wake up a lot at first, how to cope with this, and what to do to get her to sleep well in the longer term.

FOUR THINGS TO KNOW ABOUT YOUR BABY'S SLEEP:

1 | Very tiny babies wake up a lot, mainly to eat (initially about every two hours, night and day for the first couple of weeks at least).
2 | Babies sleep in 'cycles' involving periods of light dream sleep ('REM' sleep) when they twitch, flutter their eyelids and wake fleetingly, and periods of deep sleep ('non-REM' sleep) when they lie very still.
3 | Funny-sounding breathing is normal for a sleeping baby. In light sleep they can grunt, snore and have sudden intakes of breath.
4 | Almost undetectable breathing is also normal. In deep sleep they can breathe very quietly and look completely still.

So much for your baby's sleep – what about yours? Sleep deprivation can be horrendous. My second baby, Sam, was a terrible sleeper, waking up several times a night until he was over one. I spent that first year in chaos, forgetting to clean my teeth or wash the shampoo out of my hair, losing keys, pranging the car, bursting into tears and flying off the handle at the drop of a hat. Even if your sleep deprivation does not last a year, you'll still experience this to some degree because it is part of the deal for all new parents.

'You may already think your baby is sleeping like an angel. But worms can turn (and do), so don't let a peaceful eight-week-old lull you into a false sense of security.'

As your baby gets bigger, she should – in theory – start to sleep for longer and longer periods until she's going the whole night without needing you. How long it takes to achieve this Nirvana varies widely. Some babies slip seamlessly from night feeds to night-long sleeps causing their parents no heartache whatsoever. But equally, lack of sleep can be the source of huge parental angst. We think our baby 'should' be sleeping in a certain way at certain times and for certain durations, and she's not. And we have no clue what to do about it. 'The first year and a half of Rufus's life my favourite words were "should be",' says Lou, mother of two-year-old Rufus who woke up every hour and a half, night and day, until he was over one. 'We tried absolutely everything. His lack of sleep was so all-consuming it took over our lives, and put a huge strain on our relationship.'

What's the answer then? Well, if I knew, I'd be a millionaire. As Lou puts it, 'I would skim through book after book thinking, Give me the answer now! But nothing worked.' The reality is that some babies sleep well, others don't. But before you hurl yourself off Beachy Head, it's worth knowing that there *are* things you can do to encourage your baby to sleep well from day one. You may, of course, already think your baby is sleeping like an angel. But worms can turn (and do), so don't let a peaceful eight-week-old lull you into a false sense of security. Developing a good sleep strategy early in your baby's life won't be the miracle answer to all your sleep problems, but it may help.

But first, the practicalities.

HOW MUCH SLEEP DOES YOUR BABY NEED?

- An average newborn needs about sixteen and a half hours' sleep (out of twenty-four hours) in the first month. This is just an average: some need as little as twelve hours, some as many as twenty-two. Usually they'll wake every two to three hours to feed, and they may nap for less than an hour at any time. They rarely sleep for more than about four or five hours at any stretch.
- This decreases to about fifteen hours at about three months old (two-thirds of which is usually at night-time), then to fourteen and a half hours at about six months old (eleven to twelve hours at night, with a couple of daytime naps).
- Most babies will carry on having a couple of naps a day until they are about one. How long these naps last varies greatly.

In his book *Solve Your Child's Sleep Problems*, sleep expert Dr Richard Ferber says 'at some point between three and six months your baby should be sleeping well at night'. Many, obviously, aren't (hence Ferber's bestseller). If you are reading this with a tiny baby, or one that's still inside you, you may not fully appreciate the significance of getting your baby to sleep well. If you're reading this at 3 a.m., with a whisky in your trembling hand and a nine-month-old howling in the background, the penny may have dropped.

However, before you become obsessed about getting your baby to sleep well, it's important that she sleeps safely.

Sleep equipment

Essentials

- A Grobag sleeping bag appropriate for the season and your baby's size, or three to four cellular blankets *(see page 15)*. Top sheets (a sheet between baby and blanket) seem a complete waste of time, laundry and energy to me. Using a Grobag stops you worrying about all this stuff anyway.
- Three to four cotton bottom sheets (cot-sized).
- A Moses basket or crib, and from about three months a full-sized cot *(see below)*.

Handy extras

- A baby monitor, if you have a large house or garden and want to be sure you'll hear the baby. A good solid one (the UK's bestseller) is the Tomy Walkabout Classic (www.tomy.co.uk).
- A mobile or some other musical toy for the cot (a good sleep-time 'cue').
- A security object: a blankie or special toy that you always give your baby at sleep time can be really useful. You'll have to manufacture this at first – i.e. bung it next to her even when she couldn't care less. After a few months she'll start to cling to it. Ideally you want a comfort object that's washable and replaceable – a muslin square is a good idea.

What cot?

There are Rolls Royce-type cots in trendy designs, or basic Ikea models that cost very little. All are perfectly acceptable.

SOME GOOD COT FEATURES:

- It's solidly built and won't collapse.
- It has a good, preferably new, mattress that fits with no gaps and complies with British safety standards. Foam mattresses are cheaper and OK; spring or latex last longer. If you fancy a pvc-free, non-allergenic fabric try The Natural Mat Company (www.naturalmat.com). But equally, Mothercare or shops like John Lewis have a perfectly good range.
- It's convertible to a bed. Some cots will convert into a toddler bed when your baby is ready. It makes the transition easier (and cheaper) if he doesn't have to get used to an entirely new bed.

There are also a number of good sleep books – see **Contacts** for more details.

A 'Grobag' sleeping bag *(right)* keeps her snug and stops her kicking off the covers at 3 a.m. (then waking you up).

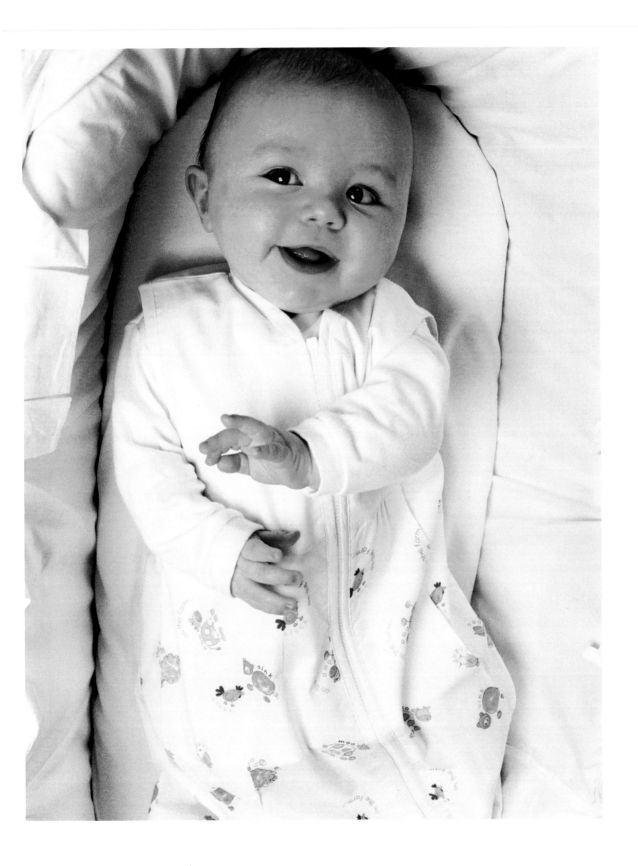

Cot death

THE FOUNDATION FOR THE STUDY OF INFANT DEATHS (FSID) SAYS:

⊙ **Cot death is more frequent in families who live in difficult circumstances or who smoke a lot.**

⊙ **Cot death is uncommon in Asian families, for reasons that are not yet understood.**

⊙ **Eighty-nine per cent of all cot deaths in England and Wales occur among babies aged under six months.**

⊙ **Cot death has fallen in the UK by seventy-five per cent since the introduction of the government's Reduce the Risk of Cot Death campaign in 1991.**

Cot death (also called Sudden Infant Death Syndrome or SIDS) is the sudden and unexpected death of a baby for no obvious reason – a huge worry to virtually all new parents. 'I was so worried about cot death I used to take her pulse in the middle of the night sometimes,' says Ginny, mother of Phoebe, nine months. Cot death is the leading cause of death in babies over one month old, which is why there's so much information about it. But it is still *rare*: in 2003 (the latest figures) there were 344 cot deaths recorded in the UK. That's 0.49 per 1,000 live births – a very small proportion.

HOW TO REDUCE THE RISK OF COT DEATH:

- Stop smoking (also in pregnancy, and this goes for dads too).
- Don't let anyone smoke in the same room as your baby.
- Always lie your baby on her back. Remember: *back to sleep*.
- Don't let your baby get too hot: if the room feels hot to you, it is to her too. Don't put on more bedding if she's unwell – a baby with a fever needs less clothing and bedding, not more.
- Keep your baby's head uncovered – put her feet at the foot of the cot (remember: *feet to foot*) so she can't wriggle down under the covers and get them over her head.
- It's safest to sleep with your baby in a cot in your bedroom for the first six months (having her in the same room as you for six months may actually slightly lower the chances of cot death).
- It's dangerous to share a bed with your baby if you or your partner:

  ⟶ are smokers (no matter where or when you smoke)
  ⟶ have been drinking alcohol
  ⟶ take medication or drugs that make you drowsy
  ⟶ feel very tired

  There is also a risk that you might roll over in your sleep and suffocate your baby, or that your baby could get caught between the wall and the bed, or could roll out of an adult bed and be injured.
- Never sleep together on a sofa, armchair or settee. This increases the risk of cot death fifty times compared with sleeping a baby in a cot in your room.
- If your baby is unwell, get medical advice as soon as you can.

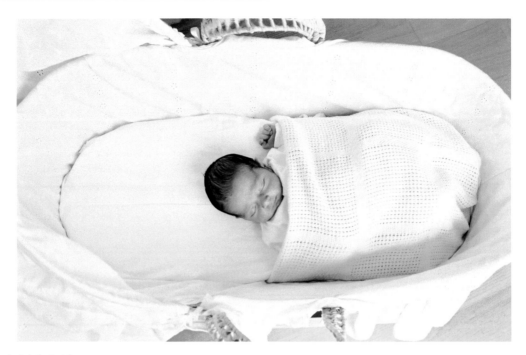

Always put your baby's feet at the bottom of the cot or Moses basket. That way, if you are using blankets, she won't shuffle down under her covers and smother herself.

IN ADDITION TO THESE ESSENTIALS, THERE ARE SOME OTHER IMPORTANT SLEEPING RULES:

- Don't give a pillow or duvet to a baby under the age of one (pillows can smother, duvets overheat).
- Don't give your baby a hot water bottle or electric blanket (there is a likelihood of overheating, burns and scalds).
- Don't let your baby fall asleep propped up on a cushion on a sofa or armchair (she could fall off, even if she's very teeny).
- Make sure the mattress fits the cot with no gaps (your baby could fall through, or get trapped or hurt).

The temperature of your baby's room should be about 16–20°C (61–68°F), but try not to get your knickers in a twist: if it's warm enough for you to be comfortable wearing light clothes, it's about the right temperature.

TO CHECK THAT YOUR BABY IS AT THE RIGHT TEMPERATURE:

To find out more about cot death, see **Contacts**.

- Touch her skin – the belly or back is best – to see if it feels hotter or colder than your skin.
- Give her one more layer of clothing (or bedding) than you're wearing, and use a Grobag appropriate for the season.
- If the room feels hot to you, keep her clothes and bedding light. In the hot summer she may only need a Babygro and a sheet.
- Don't get obsessed – just use your common sense.

Getting your baby to sleep through the night

Sleeping well is a relative concept when you become a parent. Once you've survived the first few weeks with a newborn, four uninterrupted hours of sleep on a lumpy sofa with earplugs in suddenly becomes bliss. A feed at midnight, then again at 5 a.m., is what most new parents, in the first few months, class as 'sleeping through the night'. It's hardly a lie-in. Eventually, thank the Lord, your baby should sleep continuously for around twelve hours a night. There are various things you can do to encourage this.

Swaddling

Until they are about six to eight weeks old, many babies love the feeling of being 'swaddled' – wrapped tightly in a thin cellular blanket or sheet. Swaddling can help them sleep longer as they won't wake themselves by jerking their arms or legs, and they'll feel 'safer'. Swaddled babies don't need extra blankets – make sure your baby does not get hot or sweaty. Some babies hate being swaddled, but it's probably worth a try.

How to tell if your baby is tired

It sounds obvious, but it's a key to sleep success. Look out for your baby becoming irritable or wailing, yawning, having swollen or reddish eyes or drooping eyelids. Some babies get very fretful and physically 'busy' when tired, others are more obviously dozy. Watch carefully so you get to know your baby's individual signs.

When 'should' your baby start 'sleeping through the night'?

Most babies, by around six months (and often earlier) are physically capable of getting through the night without a feed. But it doesn't mean they'll want to. If your baby is six months or older and is still waking for night feeds, it may be one of several factors:

- She's not getting enough calories in the day – make sure she has a good feed at least every three hours in the daytime. Talk to your health visitor or GP to establish whether your baby is eating enough during the day if she's waking up at night beyond six months or so, apparently ravenous.

HERE'S HOW TO SWADDLE YOUR BABY

1 | Lie your baby on a cot sheet or a cellular blanket (depending on the temperature – be very careful not to overheat her) that you have folded into a triangle shape. Her neck should be in the middle of the longest edge of the triangle, and the point should be under her feet.

2 | Hold her right arm by her side and pull the sheet over her body.

3 | Gently tuck the corner of the sheet under her left buttock.

4 | Hold her left arm down by her side.

5 | Pull the sheet over her body and tuck it under her right buttock.

6 | If the bottom of the sheet is crumpled up, straighten it. She'll look like a little mummy.

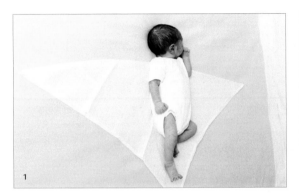

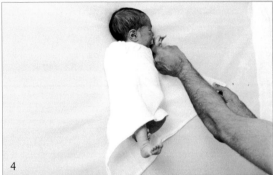

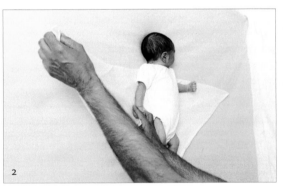

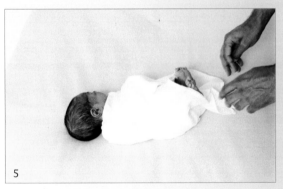

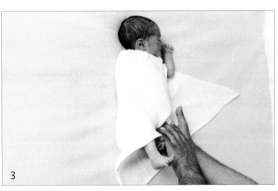

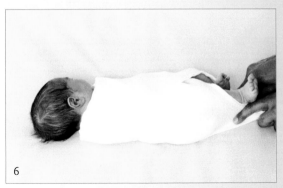

- She's in the habit of waking for comfort more than food (if this is the case, she will probably have hardly any milk before dropping off again). Try offering less and less milk, until you're just giving her water to drink. And keep it all very boring – she may wake less when she realises it's not much fun.
- She's ready to start solid food: milk just ain't enough.

AND APART FROM FOOD, THERE ARE OTHER REASONS WHY BABIES MIGHT WAKE UP AND CRY AT NIGHT:

- She is uncomfortable: a full nappy, too-tight PJs.
- She is feeing chilly or overheated.
- She is feeling unwell. See **Chapter Nine** for signs.
- She is not getting enough exercise, light and fresh air during the day. She may have pent-up energy, so get outside more and let her kick, crawl and burn it off as much as possible during the day.
- She is not getting enough naps: poor or interrupted daytime naps often mean disturbed nights.
- She may have indigestion if you've just started solids. Take weaning slowly.

How to establish good sleep habits

In the first few weeks there's nothing you can do to stop your baby waking you up a lot: she'll need to feed, be cuddled and have nappy changes, and she won't know the difference between night and day. But later on she should start to sleep for longer periods until she no longer needs you at night. Experts say that one common reason older babies wake and cry in the night (beyond illness, hunger or teething) is that they have not yet learned to put themselves back to sleep without their parents' 'help' when they wake up in their light sleep phases. Most agree that if you can help your baby, from relatively early on, to learn how to fall asleep without you, you are likely to have more peaceful nights than if she needs you to come in and sing 'Baa Baa Black Sheep' forty-eight times before she'll nod off again. They differ, of course, on exactly how to achieve this, but most agree that from very early on you want to:

- Start to teach your baby the difference between night and day.
- Do things to ensure that she can, when she's bigger and no longer needs night feeds, learn how to fall back to sleep without you if she wakes up in the night.

'Precious' sleeping conditions

If you tiptoe around when your baby is asleep, putting notices on the front door, whispering, battening down the blackout blinds and switching off the phones, you are programming your child to need pitch dark and complete silence for sleeping. This could be a bad idea if you plan to have any sort of life. What happens if the holiday house hasn't got blackout blinds? What happens when you go to stay with friends? A relatively dark, quiet place to sleep at night is good, but obsessively precious and perfect sleep conditions can be stressful to sustain in the real world.

The difference between night and day

Though your baby is bound to wake to feed at night until she's around six months old, you can still teach her from very early on that night is different from day, and that it's not interesting or fun to be awake at night.

How? In the first six weeks or so, when she's fed and sleepy, last thing at night put her to sleep in her Moses basket or crib in your quiet, dark bedroom.

THEN, DURING ALL NIGHT FEEDS:

- Keep the lights low (off if possible).
- Talk as little as possible, and use only a boring whispery voice if you have to speak.
- Don't change her nappy unless it's pooey or leaking. If you change it, do so with as little fuss as possible.
- Put her back in her cot/Moses basket as soon as you've changed/fed and burped her (avoid rocking or jiggling her back to sleep if you can).

You should also try to establish a bedtime routine so that your baby starts to learn when it is time to go to sleep at night.

YOU ARE AIMING TO:

- Put her down at bedtime after a routine that leaves her clean, fed and dozy, but not fast asleep.
- Let her drift off to sleep on her own, without you jiggling, rocking, feeding repeatedly and comforting.
- Teach her, by doing this, that if she wakes in the night she is safe, and can happily put herself back to sleep without needing you to come in (unless, of course, she still needs a feed at night, or something is wrong).

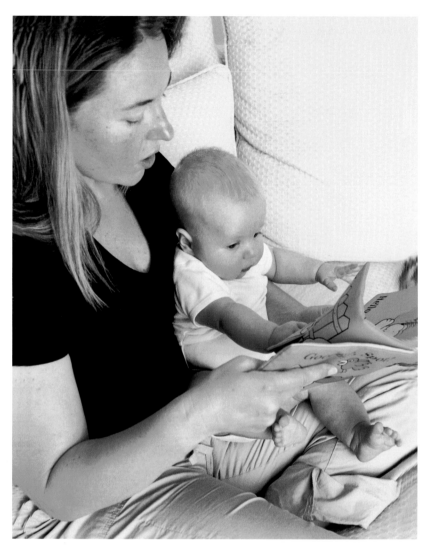

You can start giving your baby 'time for bed' signals – like having a bedtime story – from a very early age.

New babies are often up and carousing until 10 p.m. or later, but even while this phase is going on, you can teach her about bedtime by running through a lovely beddy-byes routine every night. It's a Pavlov's Dog thing: you give her a sign every night that will eventually help her to switch automatically from cavorting around to accepting that it's bedtime. For this to work you really do have to do it every night (or almost every night – if you go to a party or on holiday, a night off the routine won't hurt). As she gradually settles down more in the evenings, you can move your routine a bit earlier each night (most bigger babies – say six months and beyond – are in bed by about 6 or 7 p.m.). Initially, just do the routine around the time your baby usually falls asleep at night, even if she'll wake for a feed a few hours later.

For example, when she is starting to get sleepy and ready for bed:

- Change the 'tone' of the day: go all quiet, calm and soothing (even if your baby is yelling).
- Give her a bath, a clean nappy and some PJs.
- Feed her – in the same place every night, ideally in the bedroom where she sleeps, with only a dim light.
- Try not to let her fall asleep during the feed if you possibly can (start the routine earlier if she's crashing out every night before you get her into bed).
- Burp her and put her, *dozy but awake*, in her Moses basket/crib/cot, switch on the mobile if you have one and give her a comfort object *(see page 70)*.
- Pat, stroke or sing – the same song every night – for a minute, then leave the room saying calmly 'Night night' (ignoring any howls, which should stop after a minute or two unless this is your first attempt).

If the crying doesn't stop after a few minutes (time yourself on your watch if you find it hard not to go and comfort her), go back in. Try burping her again, then put her down, say 'Night night' and leave the room. Keep chat, jiggling and other shenanigans to an absolute minimum.

It is actually completely normal for babies to cry for a minute or two when put in bed. They're winding down, making the transition (and wondering if you'll come back). If you have eliminated as many of your concerns as possible – you've watched for signs of tiredness and know it is 'bedtime' for your baby, you've followed your routine and made sure she's had a good feed and a good burp, and you've ruled out signs of illness – you should be able to reassure yourself that it is fine for her to cry for a moment or two. As a general rule, if your baby is really distressed for more than a few minutes (five, say), I'd go back in, briefly.

If you wait to start all this until your baby is bigger – say six months plus – and is still waking up a lot at night, the learning curve can be significantly tougher. There are endless variations on how to get an older baby to sleep better at night, but probably the best known is 'controlled crying' where you let your baby cry, popping in every five minutes or so to give reassurance that you've not abandoned her, until she learns to put herself to sleep unaided. A nicer name for this general approach is 'kiss and retreat', but it can be gruelling. This is why establishing good 'sleep habits' very early on is a particularly good idea.

MOST OF US WORRY, WHEN OUR BABY CRIES AT BEDTIME, THAT:

- **She's just not tired.**
- **She's hungry.**
- **She's ill.**
- **She's in pain or discomfort.**
- **It's cruel to leave her crying, even for a moment.**
- **She's scared.**

Daytime naps

Good daytime naps tend to encourage good night-time sleeps. When they are very small, babies nap virtually all the time, but gradually some kind of pattern emerges. You might notice your baby starts to have three or four roughly consistent times of the day when she'll reliably crash out. If you follow her lead and give her the chance to nap uninterrupted at these times, this should eventually turn into a couple of decent and consistent naps (roughly a couple of hours each), one in the morning and one in the afternoon.

TO ENCOURAGE YOUR BABY TO NAP WELL, YOU NEED TO:

- Be fairly consistent once her natural napping routine has emerged – let her sleep uninterrupted at these times.
- Start to put her in her cot for these nap times.
- Start to give her a nap-time cue – not the whole bedtime routine, but something like a feed, a song, a security object, or just saying 'Nap time now', patting her and leaving the room. This can really help (Pavlov's dog again) as she gets bigger and starts to debate with you whether it is nap time or not.

Early wake-ups

At some point in the first year, some older babies suddenly start waking up horrifically early, having previously slept until 7 a.m. or later. Most of us can do anything after about 6 a.m., but 5 a.m.? Really – it's beyond the call of duty.

HERE ARE SOME THINGS TO TRY:

- Make sure the curtains really keep out the morning light. This is one instance in which blackout blinds can be a lifesaver.
- Reduce the length of her daytime naps slightly to see if it makes a difference.
- Leave her for a few minutes: many babies wake, cry, then get bored and start to play and babble to themselves, or just go back to sleep. If she's not actively howling, I wouldn't go in myself.
- If you do get up with her, keep it *very* boring (no nice stories, fun games or *Teletubbies*) – 5 a.m. = dull, dull, dull.
- If you can, avoid giving her breakfast or milk (give her water only) until her usual breakfast time, or she'll soon be waking up at 5 a.m. *because* it's breakfast time.

You

A FEW OTHER SURVIVAL TIPS:

- ⊙ **Nap whenever you can – an hour of shut-eye can make a huge difference to your sanity.**

- ⊙ **Get help so you can nap without having to cook, clean, rush to the shops or lie tensely waiting for your baby to wake up.**

- ⊙ **Take it in turns with your partner to get a 'good' night occasionally, or a lie-in.**

- ⊙ **Eat well – this can really make a difference to your energy.**

- ⊙ **Talk to someone – your health visitor, GP, other new parents or a helpline – if it's all too much.**

Books – including this one – full of 'how to get your baby to sleep advice' tend to make it all sound straightforward: do this, and this will follow. But in the real world it is often *not* that simple. Some babies *do* take longer than others to establish a routine, or never seem to get one at all. Things like illness or teething or family holidays or parental desperation or your simple lack of confidence that you're doing the right thing get in the way. Sleep problems can be hard to unravel, and many babies just never seem to sleep when, where or how they 'should'. The one thing to bear in mind is that one day your baby will be a teenager and you will be cursing her to wake up. But for now, if you're not coping, try asking your health visitor or GP if they can refer you to a sleep clinic where professionals will help you to help your baby to sleep better.

A word about selective male deafness

Some – but let me hastily add not all – dads become deaf at night. One recent survey brightly reported how fifty per cent of new dads get up in the night. I'm sorry, but what on earth do the other fifty per cent think they are playing at? You're supposed to be in this together, as a family. Even with a breastfeeding baby, a dad can give a bottle of expressed milk, change a night-time nappy, bring the baby to her mother for a feed and settle her afterwards from time to time.

> 'The one thing to bear in mind is that one day your baby will be a teenager and you will be cursing her to wake up.'

The argument that the man has to go to work and should therefore be insulated from all wake-ups is *complete rubbish*. Having one person in sole charge of all night-time wake-ups is a potentially self-destructive strategy: it frequently results in a shattered, desperate, depressed and often resentful mother alone all day in charge of a small baby – an extremely bad combination for all concerned.

Equally, if you're both up all night, you are both quickly going to become unhinged. 'We learned very early on that two sleep-deprived adults resulted in grumpy parents snapping at each other,' says Amanda, mother of Charlotte, six months. 'Therefore we ensured that only one of us was ever tired. If one had not had enough sleep

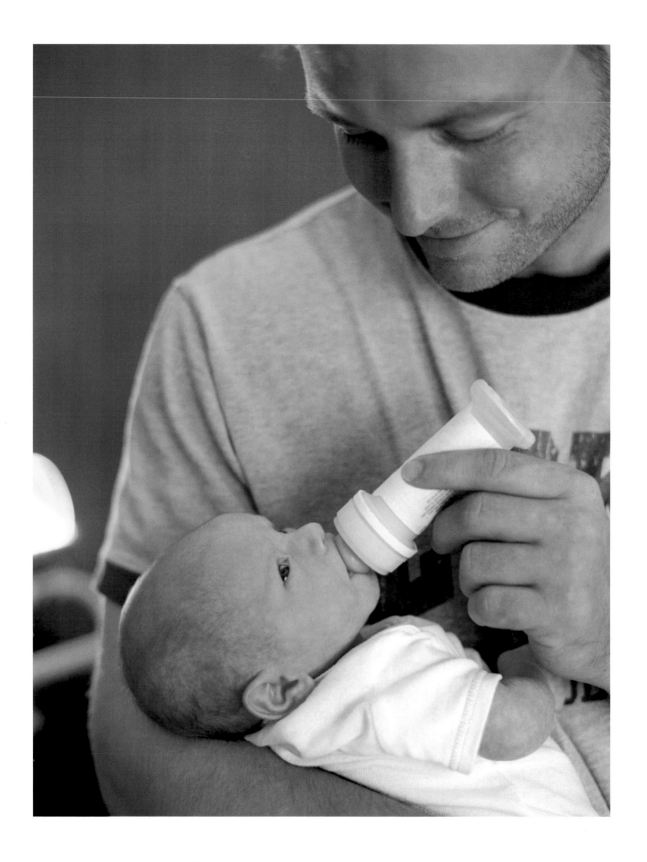

one night, the following day/night he or she was relieved of baby duty as much as possible. Even when it was me, Ian would bring Charlotte to me for feeding in the night, then take her away again as soon as she had finished.'

Sleep deprivation can do terrible things to even the most loving couple, but there are ways to get through this and still be speaking at the end of it – see **Chapter Ten**.

Lone parents: how to cope

See **Contacts** for more information on where to get help.

If you're a lone parent, this kind of debate is really going to get up your nose. Lone parents have to do *all* the night feeds, wake-ups and nappies. This is genuinely exhausting. Sorting out some kind of support network so that you can get a nap and a break in the daytime is crucial. If your family and friends aren't up to it, talk to your health visitor to find ways to get the support you really do need.

And finally, for desperate housewives ...

OK, you've read all the good sleep theory, but sometimes you're just so damned desperate you don't care any more about what you 'should' be doing. Here are some things we've all tried at some point:

- White noise. Put the Moses basket or car seat next to something like a washing machine or Hoover (some people put it on top of the dryer: only safe if you're sure – *really sure* – it can't possibly slide off).
- Sleeping tapes. Playing her tapes of 'womb-like' sounds like heartbeats, or a tape of you both talking quietly, may work.
- Use the sling. Walking, dancing or doing 'tasks' with the baby in a sling can bring instant sleep.
- Play music or the radio. Noise can actually be surprisingly soporific for a baby.
- Drive. We've all been there, bleary-eyed, at 2 a.m. on the ring road. Falling asleep at the wheel would, of course, be a very bad idea, so don't get into the car if you're really on the brink of exhaustion yourself.

There's nothing to stop dads from giving some night-time feeds from a bottle. *(left)*

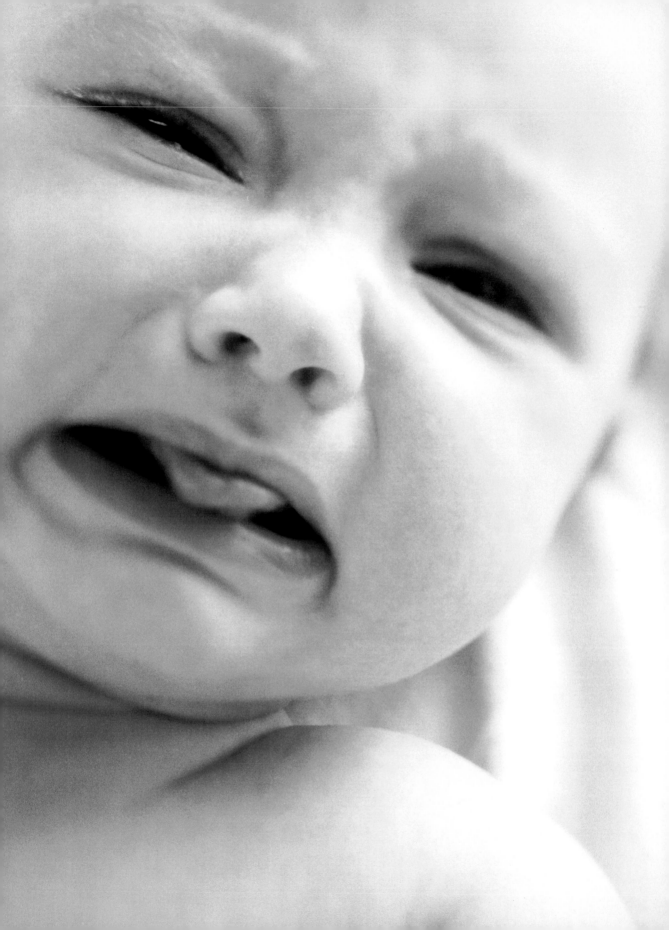

cry

Why oh why? And what to do

The chances are that when your baby is crying you're not going to be feeling entirely calm and rational. In fact, if your baby is crying a lot, you're likely to be feeling distinctly bonkers (and, potentially, anxious: what's *wrong* with him?) There are many things you can do to comfort your crying baby and prevent yourself from becoming unhinged while you do so. But the one thing to bear in mind is that babies need a lot of love, help and reassurance and, initially, they don't have many ways to tell you this beyond: 'Wah! Wah!' So brace yourself, and read on for more tips, explanations and coping strategies.

All babies cry

Some cry a *lot*. Put yourself in your new baby's position: he can't talk; he can't move much; he has no idea what's going to happen next, or whether he'll like it when it does. Crying is his only way to communicate with you. Despite this, we've somehow become conditioned to believe babies *shouldn't* cry. Crying is bad. It's somehow dangerous, 'antisocial', worrying. We, the parents, are to blame. We should be able to stop our baby crying. If we can't, we're inept. Or possibly negligent.

A baby's cry can be really hard to handle. 'Look upon crying as conversation rather than an irritant' suggests one well-meaning baby book. Fantastic advice in theory, but in practice not quite so easy. Babies cry for tons of reasons, and you may be able to work out why yours is doing so at a given time. But equally there may be no discernable reason whatsoever. The sound of your crying baby can be heart-rending, worrying, soul-destroying or infuriating. Most of the time you'll just want it to stop. Sometimes you will work out ways to soothe your baby, but not always. This is going to sound terribly selfish, but a large part of coping with your baby crying is coping with the effect the crying has on *you*.

'The sound of your crying baby can be heart-rending, worrying, soul-destroying or infuriating. Most of the time you'll just want it to stop.'

The first thing to remember is that it's not your fault – in general – that your baby is crying. Some parenting manuals give you the impression that if you do the 'right' thing at the exact 'right' time, consistently, your baby will become angelic and rarely let out a peep. This is hogwash. Some manuals instruct you to 'tap into' your baby's cry – to get to *know* that cry and what it means. This may work eventually, but in my experience when your baby's howling it's normal in the early days to feel panic and self-doubt and to be entirely unable to distinguish a 'hungry' cry from a 'fussy' cry or a 'pick me up' cry.

Most small babies just need a lot of physical comfort – they need to know, on a primitive level, that you are there, and love them, and are not going to leave them exposed on a hilltop. This existential angst may account for some of the apparently motiveless crying a small baby does. If in doubt, cuddle, cuddle, cuddle.

Calm daddies

Mothers in particular are hard-wired to respond with urgency to our baby's cries. This might be handy if there's a sabre-toothed tiger approaching, or to make sure you actually bother to put your infant to your prehistoric breast, but it can sometimes be counter-productive in the modern world. If you have adrenaline surging through your veins as you belt out 'Twinkle Twinkle Little Star', you may not be the most calming influence. The feel of a big, calm daddy who is prepared to watch footie re-runs in the wee-hours, and who is potentially less bothered by the cries, can be deeply comforting for a baby. Many fathers say they feel huge, nostalgic fondness for their 3 a.m. newborn-comforting stints. Understandably, this approach has its limits: some dads won't take kindly to being dumped with the baby every time he's crying. But finding ways to share the comforting, at different times of the day and night, is definitely a good idea.

Lone parents

Again, if you are a lone parent you are going to want to find out my address and firebomb my house. It's not easy to cope with a crying baby, but it's significantly harder if you're unable to hand him over to a partner at 2 a.m. when you're about to crack. 'I found I reached the end of my tether quite frequently,' says Mary-Ann, mother of Chloe, now two, 'and then I'd find some more tether, somehow. In a way it was good not having to deal with another person. I could do it all my way. But at times it was very lonely and despairing.' The only answer is to try everything to keep yourself as calm as possible while the crying is happening, and do what you can to get breaks during the day.

WHY oh WHY?

The crying baby checklist

Running through a mental checklist of what might be wrong may not stop your baby crying, but it may help you feel you have a modicum of control.

Sometimes, of course, it's just not that logical. And sometimes you've lost all grasp of logic because you've been up every hour for forty-eight hours and are now officially bonkers. If this is the case, try randomly selecting a few things from the 'Sixteen things to try' list *on page 92.*

CRYING TRIGGER	WHAT TO CHECK FOR/DO ABOUT IT
Tired?	Try to leave in crib for a few minutes/rock/sing
Wet?	Check nappy/Babygro
Stinky?	Ditto
Hungry?	Try feeding again, or burping then feeding. If he won't feed he's probably not hungry
Hot?	Pink cheeks? Plainly too much clothing on? Very warm back/tummy?
Cold?	Is it chilly? What's he wearing?
In pain?	Nappy rash? Tight clothing? Something sticking into him?
Fever?	Pink cheeks? Hot forehead that doesn't cool five or so minutes after removing some blankets/clothes? Take temperature
Uncomfortable?	Change the baby's position/clothes
Bored?	Been doing nothing for too long? Try smiling, talking to him, making funny noises, tickling, holding him up in the air and going 'wee' a lot
In need of comfort?	Hold close, rock, soothe, skin-to-skin, let him hear your heartbeat
In need of activity?	If he has energy to burn, let him kick around on a mat
Er ... none of the above?	He might just want a cry for no really discernable reason

Wind

Very often babies cry because of trapped wind or a tummy ache after feeds. If he seems uncomfortable (tucking his legs up, yelling, writhing, going very red in the face, arching his back) it might be because he's taking in too much air with his milk, whether breast- or bottle-fed.

SOME THINGS TO TRY:

- Burp your baby *(see page 54).*
- Gentle pressure on the baby's tummy can help. Try lying him belly-down on your lap, or holding his belly down on your forearm and patting or rubbing his back while swaying gently, even if he's not burping.
- If you're bottle-feeding, you could try different teats and brands of bottle and formula. Talk to your health visitor or GP about this.
- If you're breastfeeding, get help: talk to a breastfeeding specialist.

The evening heebie-jeebies

Many babies in the first few weeks (and sometimes for longer) have a regular time when they just cry, fret, want to suckle constantly and can't be put down. There may be all sorts of reasons for this – over-stimulation, tiredness (yours and his), tension (yours and his), hunger (if you're breastfeeding, your milk supply may be less abundant in the evening) or 'colic'. Try keeping the lights low, noises to a minimum and, if you're breastfeeding and can face it, just letting him suckle (this can help your milk supply to increase). Having a dimly lit bath together can help, or a baby massage. It also helps if you mentally just give in to the madness, accepting that for now you don't have evenings. It's an ordeal but is unlikely to last more than about twelve weeks – which of course sounds horrendous, but is nothing in terms of the rest of your life.

Colic

'Colic' is a catch-all, non-scientific term used to describe the inconsolable crying or screaming and apparent tummy pain of an otherwise healthy young baby. The symptoms are the same as wind, only more acute and long-lived, and usually start when the baby is around three weeks old, peak at around six weeks and end by about three months. Evenings are usually the worst. A colicky baby will howl at full throttle for long periods (hours, even) most days of the week. This can be genuinely traumatic for all of you.

You can go on special baby-massage courses, but there's no great secret to it. Make sure your hands are warm, and well oiled with a little grapeseed, sunflower or olive oil. Then:

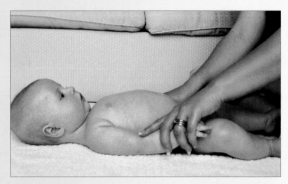

1 | Using firm but gentle strokes, place both hands on your baby's chest, massage gently upwards and outwards, over his shoulders and down his arms to his hands.

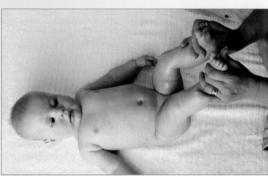

2 | Now do the length of his legs (starting from the top and moving downwards, hand over hand) and gently massage his feet.

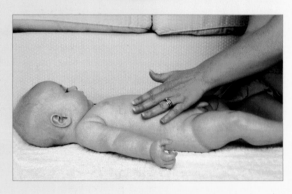

3 | Finish by gently rubbing your baby's abdomen (if your baby is newborn, you should wait until the umbilical cord has dropped off before you do this). Rubbing his tummy gently in a clockwise movement is good for tummy aches and digestion. If your baby likes it, you can then turn him over and stroke his back.

⊙ **It's not your fault.**

⊙ **It doesn't mean your baby
has a health problem.**

⊙ **It will end (usually by
twelve weeks).**

⊙ **It's not going to damage
him in the short or
long term.**

⊙ **It doesn't mean he is a
'difficult' personality.**

⊙ **It doesn't mean you're
incompetent (in fact
you're spectacular,
because you're being
pushed beyond the limits
of tolerance daily, yet are
still providing your baby
with love and care).**

Doctors don't know exactly why colic happens, but most believe
that painful gut contractions might be at least partly to blame.
Some child-rearing experts swear it is all about trapped wind.

It can be difficult to know what to do if your baby has colic.
One dad I know simply strapped the baby on to his chest in the sling
at 8 p.m. when the yelling started, put his headphones on and
listened to sport for three hours while walking round and round with
his (generally howling) baby. Another friend, Sarah, worked out a
long list of comfort techniques for her colicky baby Hazel and divided
the nightly three hours of colic time into fifteen-minute segments.
Each fifteen minutes she switched to something different. Hazel still
yelled most of the time, but Sarah swears this 'management'
approach helped her stay sane. In short, you may not be able to stop
your baby's colic, but you may be able to find a way to cope that keeps
you from losing your mind.

HERE ARE SOME OTHER THINGS TO DO:

1 | Get support. Ask your health visitor if there are any local support
groups. Serene, incorporating the Cry-Sis Helpline, is for parents
of 'excessively crying, sleepless and demanding babies and
young children'. Or you could try the NSPCC Child Protection
Helpline. They won't think you're a child abuser, 'at risk' or
anything like that – they are used to supporting 'normal' parents
with crying babies. You will find the details of both these
organisations in **Contacts**.

2 | Get practical help. Accept all the help you can get – day or night –
around the house and with your baby. Make sure that somehow,
every day if possible, you get some time out for yourself (even a
ten-minute walk alone can help).

3 | Try everything. Try all the methods, holds and tricks *(see page 92)*
to soothe babies. Something may work, even if it's just for
five minutes.

The 'crying type'

Your baby may cry more than your friend's baby. So what? What's
wrong with having a lively, communicative, sensitive baby? Many a
granny will tell you that crying is a sign of intelligence. A lot of crying
is certainly *not* a sign that you have a hyperactive/oversensitive/
attention-deficit-disordered/whingeing child. A crying baby is,
in essence, and though it might not feel that way at times,
a communicative one.

Sixteen things to try with your crying baby

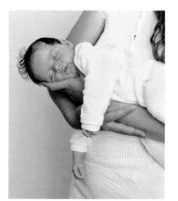

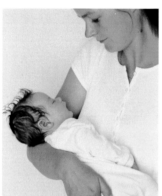

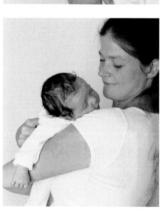

Different babies like being 'snuggled' in different ways: along your arm *(top)*, 'rockabye' style *(middle)* or upright against your shoulder *(bottom)*.

Once you've ruled out 'hard' causes like hunger, wet/dirty nappies, pain or other physical discomfort, try a few of these:

1 | Snuggle him close to your body. He's been squished up in your womb for nine months, so will probably like being held close, either upright on your shoulder, 'rockabye' style or face down on your arm (experiment with what 'hold' he likes best).

2 | Move. Gently and rhythmically bounce/jiggle/dance/sway while holding him close.

3 | Make repetitive noises. It's usually best to do this while moving. You'll sound and possibly look insane, but it can help.

4 | Play music. All three of our babies stopped crying when we played them the reggae classic 'People Funny Boy' by Lee 'Scratch' Perry that begins, bizarrely, with the sound of a baby wailing. Distraction? Rhythm? Who knows? But it's worth a go. Try anything – a friend of mine says that hardcore Belgian techno worked wonders on their baby.

5 | Try white noise. Put his Moses basket/chair by a washing machine, dryer or even a Hoover or hairdryer. Or try switching on burbling Radio 4.

6 | Let him suck your (clean) finger, or his thumb/fingers/fist, or a dummy if you are using one *(see page 94)*.

7 | Have a bath. Both of you together often works well.

8 | Hand him to someone else. They have a different vibe, not magic powers: he may simply get interested in the new face/smell/position and forget about crying.

9 | Go outside. Walk into the garden (even in winter – just grab a blanket) to give him a change of air temperature, noise, atmosphere and light.

10 | Drive. I'd use this as a last resort unless you want to spend ninety per cent of your first few weeks as a parent on the dual carriageway.

11 | Use a baby sling. Try putting him in the sling and getting on with things like the washing-up, cooking or cleaning.

12 | Sing. He heard your voice for nine months, so it's what he knows best in this loud, alien world.

13 | Give him a massage. It never worked for me – when my babies were howling, stripping them down and slathering them in oil was the last thing they wanted – *but* many, many other mothers have told me it worked wonders for them. Try a drop or two of pure lavender essential

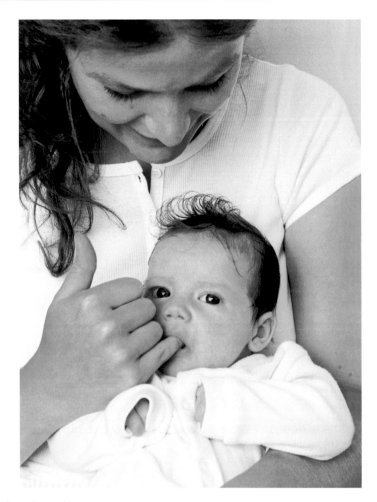

Letting your baby suck your clean finger is a great way to comfort him.

To find out more, or to find a practitioner, try the General Osteopathic Council (details in **Contacts**).

oil in a base of a pure oil like grapeseed or sunflower. Don't get too hung up on method and equipment, unless you want to. Just lie him on a warm towel in a warm room and stroke his body with soothing, firm but gentle strokes, using warm oiled hands. If he likes it, try doing his back and front.

14 | Change his nappy and clothes (even if they are clean). Occasionally I've found this will distract a crying baby. Maybe the familiarity of the changing routine helps. It can, equally, enrage them, but it's worth a go.

15 | Lie him down. It took us ages to realise this, but our third baby, Ted, often just wanted to be put down.

16 | See a cranial osteopath. Cranial osteopathy is a very subtle type of osteopathic treatment that encourages the release of stresses and tensions (incurred during the birth) throughout your baby's body. Lots of parents believe it helped their fretful babies.

At the end of your tether

Shaking

Never do it. Shaking your baby, even fleetingly, can cause bleeding in the brain that can damage, if not kill, your baby. If you feel you're losing it, *always* put him down somewhere safe and leave the room until you are calmer again.

Five things to do now before you snap

1 | Breathe. Slowly in to a count of five, expanding your abdomen, and out to a count of ten, pulling it in. Do this ten times. Try visualising yourself in a beautiful calm place as you do this (that beach in Barbados ...)

2 | Get out of earshot. Put him down in a safe place (for example his Moses basket, cot, car seat or bouncy chair), shut the door and get yourself into a different room for a short while where you can't hear him (put on the radio or some loud music if necessary). Just ten minutes' time out can pull you back from the brink. This is not bad parenting – in fact, it's good parenting. Your baby will be fine, even if he seems outraged.

3 | Phone someone. Call your mum, friend, partner or health visitor and cry if necessary. Most grandmothers have, at some point, had their child and grandchild howling at them simultaneously down the phone.

4 | Remind yourself it's not your baby's fault. He's not bad. He's not 'difficult'. He's not trying to punish you. He's just a little baby.

5 | Remind yourself it's not your fault. You're not doing it all wrong, and feeling upset, in despair or angry is not a sign that you're failing to cope. It's normal.

Dummies

What's the debate?

The pros: sucking is comforting for babies, and getting your baby to take a dummy can really help calm him when he cries (and get him to fall asleep); it can also help a small baby last a tiny bit longer between feeds, if you are trying to do this.

The cons: the World Health Organization says using dummies can interfere with breastfeeding and that they've been linked to dental problems, ear infections and stomach and mouth infections, but only usually as the baby gets bigger; there is some evidence that dummies (presumably if used a lot) can interfere with the babbling and other sounds a baby makes in preparation for speech, starting somewhere around six months; finally, if your baby can only fall asleep with a dummy, problems may arise if his dummy falls out in his sleep and he wakes (you) up wailing for it ten times a night.

Good dummy use

MANY PARENTS DECIDE:

- Only to use a dummy for six months then ditch it before dependency really kicks in
- Only to use the dummy to help him fall asleep, then take it out once he's sleeping
- To avoid using the dummy when he's awake, so there is no interference with emerging babbling sounds and conversation

However you decide to use one, make sure it is very clean (don't lick it, as you will transfer the bacteria from your mouth to the dummy). The official advice is that dummies should be sterilised for babies under six months.

Why you should respond to your baby's crying but not panic

'Spoiling' isn't an issue with a tiny baby, but loving him *is* – as is *showing him* you love him and are there for him. So you should definitely respond to your baby's cries: he needs to know he's important and loved and has not been abandoned on a hilltop for the vultures.

However, there's a big caveat here. If you are on the loo, it will not kill your baby to yell in his cot for a minute or two. If you are going nuts he will be fine howling for ten minutes while you calm down (much finer than he'd be if you yelled at him, shook him or otherwise harmed him). First babies are the only ones who get insta-mum ('n' dad) night and day. Subsequent babies all survive in a universe of delayed parental response perfectly well. Ted, my third, is the happiest one-year-old imaginable, despite frequently being left to shout while I break up a fight, feed his siblings or stop them swinging from the lampshades.

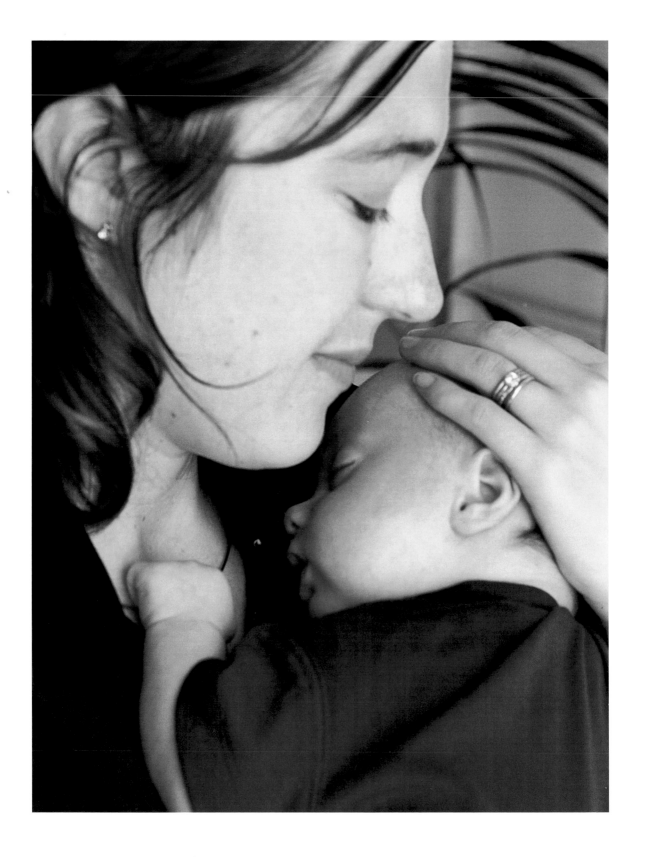

Boys don't cry

Don't go there. Studies have actually found that boy babies cry more than girl babies, and get more stressed, particularly in new situations. Don't fall into the trap of trying to 'toughen' your little lad up by leaving him unconsoled. He's a tiny baby, for goodness sake, and you want him to grow up into a nice, sensitive man, not a Neanderthal. Baby boys (like girls) cannot be 'mollycoddled'.

'Odd' crying

If your baby's crying suddenly starts to sound 'different' to you – high-pitched, wailing, whimpery or just not his usual cry, your instinct will be to pay attention. This is good. Sometimes the explanation is simple – he's just exhausted because you've had him out at a party and he's over-excited. But sometimes it's a sign that he's ill. If your baby's cry just feels 'wrong', or is making you panicky, go with your feelings and call the doctor.

Bigger babies

After about three months, other reasons for crying start to crop up:

- Anxiety. An older baby may cry because he doesn't want you to leave, he's scared of something or you've changed something (like his room or his routine). One good rule is always to say 'goodbye' before you leave him with someone. Even if you are just popping to the loo, say, 'Bye-bye, Mummy's coming back in a minute.' It may make him cry more in the instant, but if he knows you'll always tell him when you're leaving, he won't be constantly anxious that you're going to sneak off when his back is turned.
- Frustration. Older babies can get fussy around their physical 'milestones': a baby who wants to crawl, but can't, may for a few weeks become incredibly grumpy every time you put him down.
- Fears. After about six months babies often seem to become more frightened of 'new' things – like a loud lorry, a mooing cow, a clown or a big balloon. Reassurance, cuddles and comfort are, in general, a better idea than forcing your baby to face something that scares him.

See **Contacts** for good books on dealing with colicky/crying babies.

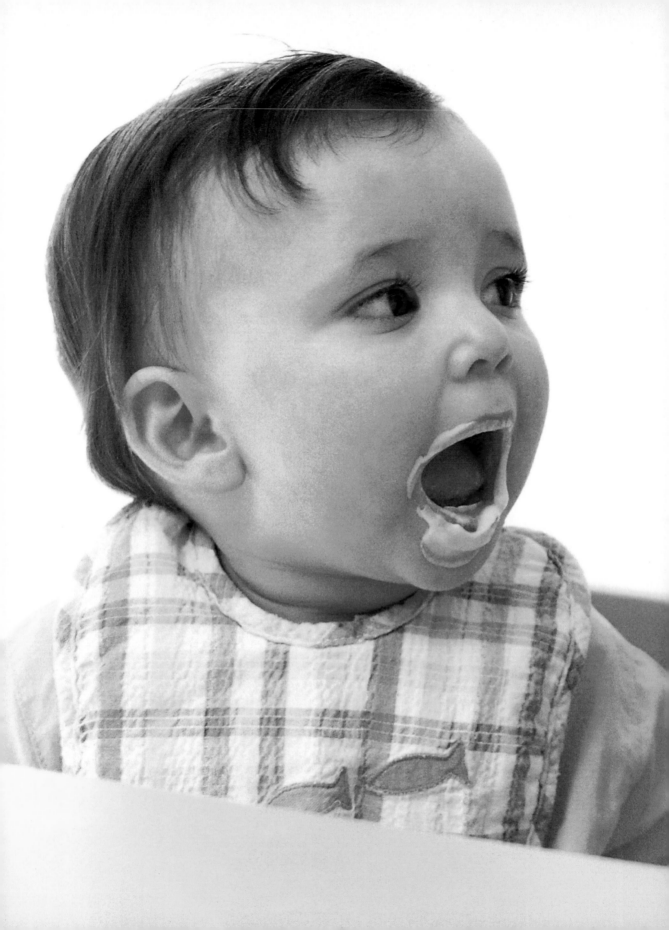

eat

Feeding your baby from day one to family mealtimes

Your baby, like you, is an individual. Sometimes she'll be hungry, sometimes not. Sometimes peckish. Occasionally ravenous. And sometimes she'll just fancy a comfort snack. Feeding your baby is not, then, simply about fuel. Nor should it be done with military precision. It can't be. Food (milk included) is about love, reassurance, pleasure, habits and – when you consider the amount of farting, burping, pooing and throwing up that goes on – the odd bit of pain. It can take a while to get the hang of feeding and then, just as you've cracked it, it's time for solids – a whole new ball game.

Breastfeeding

Breast milk is a wonderful invention. It provides all the nutrition your baby needs for the first six months, reduces her risk of developing gastroenteritis, eczema, childhood diabetes and respiratory, urinary tract and ear infections; it may lower her risk of developing childhood leukemia; and it certainly lowers your risk of developing pre-menopausal breast cancer and ovarian cancer. It's also handy: you can breastfeed anywhere and it takes no preparation. Even if you only manage to breastfeed for a few weeks, your baby can benefit. But if you can possibly keep it up for six months, or even a year, you've done fantastically.

How does it work?

Your baby's sucking sends messages to your brain that tell the ducts in your breasts to contract and eject milk. When your baby is born, your breasts produce their first food: colostrum. This contains sugar, protein, antibodies and hormones. One to four days after the birth, but sometimes longer (particularly if you've had a Caesarean), your milk will 'come in'. Most (but not all) women find their breasts get really swollen and obviously 'full' when this happens. Gradually this 'supply and demand' starts to balance out and feeds become more regular.

Is it easy?

Although about seventy per cent of us start off breastfeeding our babies, one fifth give up within the first two weeks and over a third of us have stopped by the time the baby is six weeks old. Ninety per cent of women who give up breastfeeding within six weeks say they'd have liked to breastfeed for longer. So the answer to this question for many women is a resounding no. As Sally Inch, who runs the breastfeeding clinic at the Oxford Radcliffe Hospitals NHS Trust puts it, 'Breastfeeding is a learned skill. It's natural but not instinctive.'

YOU'RE DOING IT RIGHT IF:

- It doesn't hurt.
- Your baby suckles almost immediately.
- Her sucking pattern changes from quick short sucks to slow deep sucks.
- She is relaxed throughout.
- She pauses from time to time, then starts again without having to be coaxed.

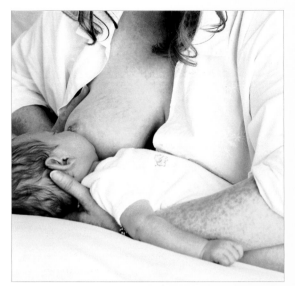

HOW TO LATCH YOUR BABY ON PROPERLY

This is the major key to breastfeeding success.

1 | Get comfortable in a chair that supports your back, or lying on your side on a sofa or bed. You should be able to hold your baby close to your breast without straining. If you're sitting, try raising your legs on a footstool or a couple of phone books (tape them together with masking tape). You might want to put your baby on a pillow or two if she's on your lap.

2 | Position your baby with her nose – not her mouth – opposite your nipple before you start to feed. Hold her body so that she can come up to your breast from below (you're going to bring her to your breast, not the other way round). Her top eye should be able to make eye contact with you.

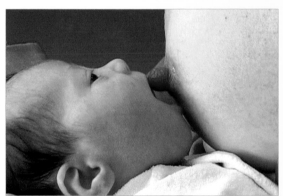

3 | Encourage your baby to open her mouth really wide (gape). Brush her top lip against your nipple to get her mouth to open widely and, as she drops her lower jaw, bring her towards your breast fairly quickly. Let her head tilt backwards as you do this, so her chin and lower jaw reach your breast first. Aim her lower lip as far away from the base of your nipple as possible: this way she can scoop in a deep mouthful of the breast tissue below the nipple too. This is your key to success. Remember, as breastfeeding specialists say, it's breastfeeding, not nipple-feeding.

4 | Try again if it hurts. It's normal for it to hurt fleetingly but if, beyond the first few sucks, it keeps hurting, she's not latched on right (or there may be some other problem, *see page 104*). Put one of your fingers into her mouth gently to break the suction, take her off and try again. Keep trying until it feels more comfortable.

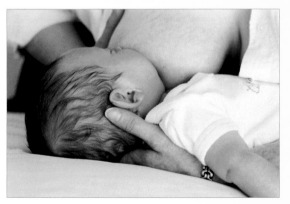

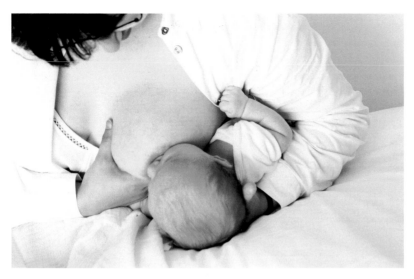

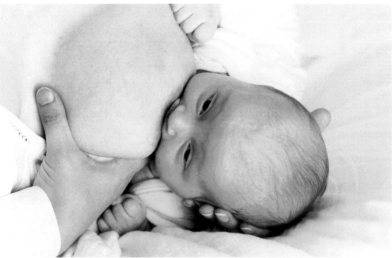

Try different positions – the 'rugby hold' *(shown above)* is great for post-Caesarean recovery.

- She can breathe without you having to press the breast away from her nose.
- Her chin is touching your breast.
- Her mouth looks wide open.
- Should you be able to see any of the dark bit around your nipple (the areola), the visible bit is above her top lip, not below the bottom one (get someone to look for you).
- She lets go spontaneously when she's done (or lets go when you gently raise the breast).
- When she comes off the breast your nipple is the same shape as it was when she started (if it looks squashed it was not far back enough in her mouth).

How often, how long?

The randomness and relentlessness of early breastfeeding surprises most women. It can be genuinely exhausting.

THESE ARE THE BASIC RULES FOR THE FIRST FEW WEEKS:

- Feed your baby whenever she seems to want it.
- Feed her for however long she wants to feed.
- Offer both breasts at every feed, but only once she comes off the first breast. If you swap her from one breast to the other too soon, she may only be getting the thinner 'fore milk' from each breast. The 'hind milk' that comes later in a feed is richer and has more calories, so you want her to stay on until she's getting this.
- After the first week, when feeds will be very frequent, aim to feed her about six to eight times in twenty-four hours. But remember her timing is unlikely to be completely consistent, though it should get gradually more predictable.

Other drinks

Before about six months when you start weaning, your fully breastfed baby doesn't need additional drinks – including water – unless the doctor advises it. Bottle-fed babies can be offered cooled boiled water as an extra drink in hot weather.

Dads and breastfeeding

Studies show that dads are key to breastfeeding success. Your partner may appear to do very little for the first week or so other than feed the baby. This may look relaxing, but it may feel exhausting and overwhelming to her. You can help on a practical level by bolstering her with encouragement and allowing her to rest.

HERE'S HOW:

- Sometimes be the one to get your baby out of the Moses basket/ cot during the night and hand her over for feeds or change a pooey nappy so that your partner is not always having to get up.
- During the day take the baby off her hands sometimes between feeds so she gets a break.
- Bring your partner things she needs while breastfeeding (drinks, snacks, remote control) – she may feel trapped sitting in a chair for long periods.

The main reasons we stop before we want to

LACK OF CONFIDENCE

Nearly half of us give up in the early stages because we think we don't have enough milk. This is actually immensely rare (even if you have twins). Whether or not your breasts feel 'full' is no indication of whether they are producing enough milk, and size doesn't matter: tiny boobs can produce vast quantities of milk. It can, however, take a while to build up both your confidence and your milk supply (particularly for evening feeds when you're knackered). If your baby has plenty of wet nappies every day (ten or so) and is growing according to the Breast from Birth charts *(see below)*, she is getting enough milk.

UNPREDICTABILITY OF FEEDS

In the early days your baby might not feed for four hours, then may feed every hour for a bit. A feed can last anything from ten minutes to an hour, and can be one breast or both. You may feel you do virtually nothing but feed the baby. This can undermine your confidence if you're expecting regular three-hourly schedules.

'BREAST PROBLEMS'

Anything from sore nipples to mastitis (inflammation of the breast tissue) can knock you for six. See the **Troubleshooting** section below.

UNHAPPY BABY

Get some specialist breastfeeding help if your baby is:

- Not coming off the breast spontaneously after she's fed
- Restless or writhing as she feeds
- Not satisfied after a long feed
- Very windy or uncomfortable after feeding
- Taking a long time (if latched on well, most feeds take between five and thirty minutes per breast)
- Feeding very frequently (more than ten feeds in twenty-four hours after the first few days)
- Hardly feeding at all (fewer than three feeds in the first twenty-four hours and fewer than six feeds in twenty-four hours when one to two days old)
- Still doing black poos when she's thirty-six to forty-eight hours old

Troubleshooting: some common problems

CONFUSED ABOUT TECHNIQUE?

Every midwife and health visitor can appear to have a different 'solution'. The breastfeeding part of their training is currently very variable, so the advice they give may be inconsistent and conflicting. By all means try things they suggest, but talk to an infant-feeding specialist if problems persist.

BABY NOT GAINING ENOUGH WEIGHT

The weight chart that your health visitor has may not apply to your baby. It may be based on data from (largely Caucasian), formula-fed babies. Breastfed babies tend to gain weight, perfectly healthily, at a different rate from formula-fed ones – usually quicker in the first couple of months, then slowing up around two to three months. When this happens, many health visitors suggest 'supplementing' feeds with formula: this is the quickest way to scupper your breastfeeding. If your health visitor suggests supplementing feeds:

- Ask if she is using the Child Growth Foundation's Breast from Birth chart – if not, ask her to get hold of one.
- Try to increase your milk supply *(see below)*.
- Talk to an infant-feeding specialist about your technique.

FOUR WAYS TO INCREASE YOUR MILK SUPPLY

1 | Make sure your baby is latched on properly.
2 | Feed 'on demand', not according to some rigid schedule.
3 | Try getting into bed with your baby, ideally skin-to-skin, and staying there for twenty-four hours, just feeding whenever she wants (put her in her cot or Moses basket next to you when you are sleeping).
4 | Feed more frequently: could you fit in an extra feed or two in twenty-four hours? The more you feed the more your breasts produce.

In a sense, a vital part of breastfeeding success is to let go of your preconceptions – and desire for control. Forget about schedules and timing and amounts: just feed your baby when she seems interested. Feeding your baby isn't just about fuel. As UNICEF breastfeeding expert Sue Ashmore puts it: 'Breast milk is far more than food or drink for a baby. It is comfort, attention and love too.'

ENGORGED BREASTS

They can become very hard, flushed, painful and full, usually in the early days of feeding. If your baby is emptying the breast well at every feed, engorgement should be a very temporary thing. But for countless women it isn't.

The way to deal with this is to increase the amount of milk that is removed from your breasts and improve how your baby is latching on. Some health professionals will tell you that if you remove milk with a breast pump, you will make the problem worse because your breast will then produce even more milk. This is not true. Gently using a breast pump after a feed is very useful for engorged breasts. You could also try expressing a small bit of milk before a feed (during a warm bath or shower is easiest). This can help it hurt less when your baby latches on. Because she's getting a better mouthful of breast, it can help her latch on more easily too. Get a specialist to check your latch-on technique.

Studies show that putting Savoy cabbage leaves on your breasts (a common 'remedy' for engorgement) has no real effect: the coldness may soothe your breasts, but cabbage leaves won't sort out the real problem, which is removing milk from the breast efficiently.

SORE/CRACKED/BLEEDING NIPPLES

Nipples can be torture but, though incredibly common, this is not 'normal': it is usually a sign that your latch-on technique is not working well.

IF YOU HAVE PAINFUL NIPPLES, YOU SHOULD:

- Get an infant-feeding specialist to help you latch your baby on correctly.
- Keep feeding, or express milk using a pump if feeding is too sore and feed it to your baby in a bottle.
- Avoid putting any soaps, creams or lotions on to your nipples.
- Try putting Vaseline or a lanolin-based cream on to soothe them (Lanisoh is a great product).

THRUSH

Sometimes sore nipples are caused by a yeast infection ('thrush') in your nipple and the baby's mouth. The signs are bright pink and tender nipples, and shooting pains while breastfeeding and between feeds. Your baby may have white patches in her mouth (these look like milk curds that won't wipe off). See your GP for simple thrush treatment for you and your baby.

MASTITIS AND 'BLOCKED DUCTS'

Mastitis is an *inflammation* of the breast tissue (it is rarely an 'infection'), almost always caused by the breast not being emptied thoroughly by your baby when she feeds (that latch-on again). It usually begins with lumpy areas on the breast but not much pain (this is often called a 'blocked duct'). If the milk stays in this blocked duct, the pressure rises, forcing the milk through the lining of your milk ducts and into the surrounding breast tissue, where it causes an acute inflammation inside the breast, which turns red, hot and very painful. If this milk then enters your bloodstream, you start to feel fluey – your immune system is treating the milk as if it were a foreign protein.

'Nipples can be torture but, though incredibly common, this is not 'normal': it is usually a sign that your latch-on technique is not working well.'

As soon as you suspect you have a blocked duct, you should see an infant-feeding specialist – the same day if at all possible. Most GPs mistakenly think of mastitis as an 'infection' and prescribe antibiotics, but though they are anti-inflammatory, and therefore helpful, they won't cure the problem. Many breastfeeding helplines tell you to put flannels on the breast and massage it, but this, says Sally Inch, who also happens to be author of the World Health Organization briefing on mastitis 'is missing the point, and may on occasions make the problem worse'. Latching your baby on right, so that she can remove milk efficiently at each feed, is vital.

WHILE YOU'RE WAITING TO GET HELP WITH YOUR TECHNIQUE

- Keep feeding your baby, even though it will hurt a lot.
- Take maximum doses of ibuprofen (it reduces inflammation and pain).
- Use a breast pump after each feed (to ensure that the milk is moving through your breast even if the baby isn't latched on well).

FEELING SELF-CONSCIOUS ABOUT FEEDING

In a society that loves nothing more than Jordan's boobs, it's a little bizarre that a glimpse of a breast doing what it is actually designed for should be greeted with disapproval. Still, the first few times you breastfeed in a public place, you may feel as if you're in one of those nightmares where you're running naked down Oxford Street.

HOW TO COPE:

- Remember it is perfectly legal to breastfeed in public.
- Try draping a blanket over your shoulder and baby while she feeds.
- Keep doing it: the more you do it, the more comfortable you'll become.

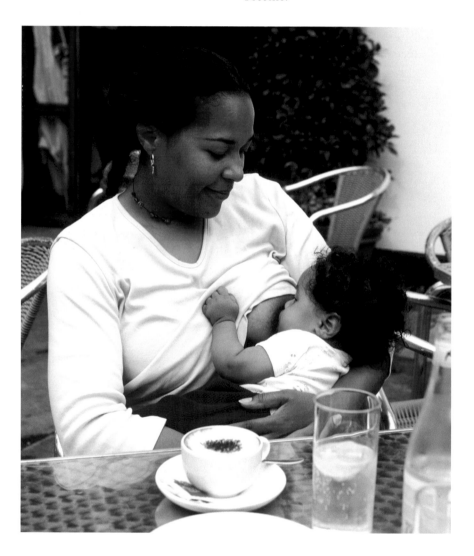

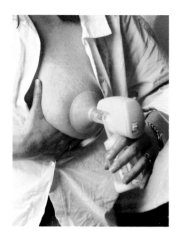

A FEW HYGIENE TIPS:

- **Express your milk into a sterilised bottle using a sterilised pump.**

- **Put the milk straight into the fridge.**

- **Only keep it in the fridge for twenty-four hours.**

- **If you freeze it, do so soon after pumping (you can buy special sterile freezer bags for breast milk). It will keep frozen for up to six months.**

- **Defrost the milk in the fridge, then use it within twelve hours.**

See **Contacts** for more details on where to get help with breastfeeding.

- Avoid shirts that unbutton, making you feel naked. T-shirts and tops you can pull up discreetly work best. Those silly breast-feeding tops with enormous 'pockets' are not only a fashion crime, they're pointless.

- Bigger branches of some shops (such as Boots, Sainsbury's and Debenhams) have mother and baby rooms. Some county councils also produce a guide to smoke-free places to eat, and some include details on whether a place 'welcomes' breastfeeding mothers.

IF IT DOESN'T WORK OUT

If you've set your heart on breastfeeding, but can't, it can be tough to get out the formula. 'I felt like I was feeding him poison when I first gave him a bottle,' says Gemma, mother of Luca, two. 'I'd wanted desperately to breastfeed, but he just wouldn't do it. I still feel sad about it.' While studies show that breastfeeding is 'best' for babies (and mothers), this does not mean the bottle is bad. Infant formula is nutritionally perfectly adequate for most babies, so try not to beat yourself up if you aren't able to continue breastfeeding.

How to express milk

Expressing some milk into a bottle using a breast pump or your hands (so your baby can sometimes be fed by someone else) is a handy skill. But it can also feel frustrating, weird and sometimes very, very slow. Get your midwife or health visitor to show you how to express at first. The usual advice is to wait until your baby is around six weeks old and your milk supply has settled down a bit before trying to express, but there's no reason not to start earlier if you want or need to. I'd try it first thing in the morning: you're likely to have the most milk then.

It's best to try feeding your baby expressed milk in a bottle before she's about eight weeks because it can be really hard to get bigger babies to take a bottle *(see page 114)*.

Where to go for help

If you're having any problems, always try to get to a breastfeeding clinic or an infant-feeding specialist as soon as you possibly can. If your hospital does not have a breastfeeding clinic or 'lactation specialist', there are a number of organisations that can help, including La Leche League, the National Childbirth Trust, the Breastfeeding Network and the Association of Breastfeeding Mothers.

Bottle-feeding

Though it doesn't involve any physical pain, bottle-feeding has its ups and downs too. Here are the essentials, but the best place to go for more help with bottle-feeding issues is your midwife or health visitor.

How often, how much?

The general and, I'd say, sensible advice is to feed 'on demand': in the first few days this may be every hour or two (about 45 ml (1 1/2 fl oz) at a time). By two or three weeks, your baby might last two to three hours between feeds. Ultimately most bottle-fed babies settle into a routine of feeding every three hours or so, but certainly at first just make up a bottle if you think she might be hungry, even if it's only a little while since the last feed. You're bound to make up a bottle sometimes that is rejected – just chuck it away and move on.

Until she weighs about 4.5 kg (10 lb), your baby will probably want, as a rough guide:

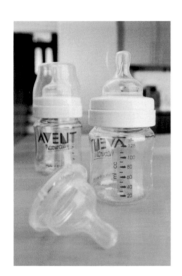

- By week one about 60 ml (2 fl oz) at each feed
- By week four about 125 ml (4 fl oz) at each feed
- By week twelve about 210 ml (7 fl oz) at each feed

But try not to get obsessed by quantity or timing: your baby will tell you how much she wants to eat and when. She'll refuse the milk when she's full (but do burp her to make sure it's not just wind that's stopping her). If she falls asleep halfway through a feed, try waking her after ten minutes or so to see if she wants to continue (try changing her nappy to wake her up). Don't try and force her to finish a bottle – it's pointless.

How to make up a bottle

It's so easy your newborn could practically do it herself:

1 | Wash your hands.
2 | Get a sterilised bottle and put in 125 ml (4 fl oz) cooled boiled water from the kettle.
3 | Add level scoops of powdered formula exactly according to the packet instructions – level each scoop off with a knife.
4 | Put the lid on and shake until the powder has dissolved.
5 | Warm to body temperature – test it on the inside of your wrist.

When bottle-feeding *(right)*, you want the teat to be full of milk, not air.

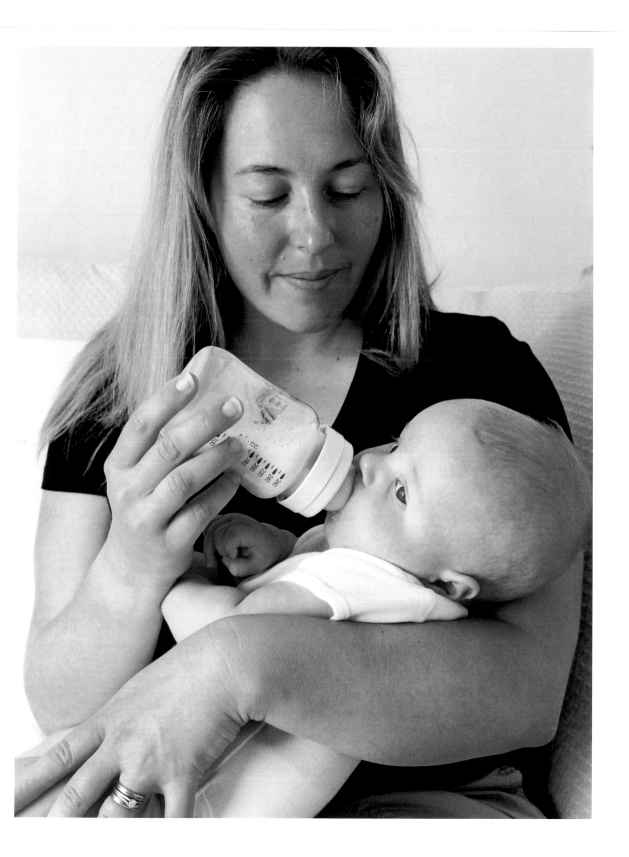

How to warm a bottle

Put the bottle (lid on) into a measuring jug or bowl of hot water for a few minutes, then test the temperature on your wrist. The official advice is not to heat bottles in the microwave because you can get 'hot pockets'. In the interests of full disclosure, I should mention here that virtually all the experienced mothers I know heat bottles of formula in the microwave (not breast milk, though, as it can be damaged by microwave heating). We heat for twenty to thirty seconds, shake the bottle very well and test it a couple of times on our wrist before feeding the baby. We will all probably be rounded up and shot at dawn for this, but I thought you should at least know the truth. Clearly the 'safest' way would be the hot-water route.

How to feed a bottle to your baby

1 | Hold her close against your body, resting in the crook of one arm as you look into her eyes: you want her to feel secure and warm.
2 | Hold the bottle like a pen, and keep it tilted so the teat is always full of milk – not air, which can make your baby windy.
3 | Let her feed for as long as she wants.
4 | Throw away unused milk, even if it's practically a whole bottle. Feeding it to her later could make her sick.
5 | If she starts writhing or crying halfway through, try burping her and offering her the bottle again.
6 | Then accept that no means no, even if you *really* want her to have more.

Keeping things clean

Bottles and teats (and your breast pump if you use one) need to be very, very clean. Wash them up with a long bottle brush, or in the dishwasher, then the general advice is to sterilise them.

YOU CAN STERILISE EQUIPMENT BY:

- Using steam sterilisers that plug in or go into the microwave
- Using sterilising tablets or Milton Fluid in which you soak your equipment
- Simply boiling or steaming the equipment using a large pan of water for ten minutes

Most experienced mothers I know use a steriliser that you pop in the microwave. We all agree this is somehow easier than the alternatives, but we don't know why.

Other bottle-feeding rules

- Keep made-up formula in the fridge. The official advice is that a bottle of formula shouldn't be out of the fridge for more than an hour.
- Throw away any formula left in the bottle after every feed – even if your baby hardly touched it.
- Use the formula before its best-before date.
- Never prop the bottle up on something to feed the baby: she could choke. (How you'd actually physically achieve this is beyond me, but if you're tempted, just don't).
- Never add anything – extra formula, rusks, baby rice – to the milk (no matter what Granny suggests). This can make your baby sick.

Night feeds

A FEW TIPS THAT CAN HELP MAKE NIGHT-TIME FEEDS EASIER FOR EVERYONE:

⊙ **Have your night-time bottles made up and ready in the fridge.**

⊙ **Keep the lights dim.**

⊙ **Keep your voice low.**

⊙ **Take it in turns with your partner to feed the baby.**

In the first eight weeks or so, most babies need a feed last thing at night (say 10 or 11 p.m.), and then another one somewhere between about midnight and 6 a.m. when they wake up hungry. Most are able to drop this middle of the night feed by the time they're eight to twelve weeks old, but some keep demanding night feeds for a very long time (see **Chapter Four**).

How to bottle-feed in the outside world

You don't need to rush home for feed time like some deranged Cinderella, nor do you have to be fussing around with ten tons of equipment. You can buy small cartons of ready-made formula (from any supermarket or places like Boots) to take out with a sterilised bottle. The milk will be room temperature and so ready to decant and feed whenever you need to.

I'm not sure why anyone would do anything else, but you can also prepare a feed to take with you. Fill a sterilised bottle with warm (not boiling – let it cool a bit) water from the kettle, then measure out the right amount of milk powder for that amount of water into a clean Tupperware container. The water cools over the next hour or so (*check the temperature before you offer it to your baby, obviously*) and you make up the bottle when you need it.

If you can get your baby to accept room temperature (or even cold) milk, life is a breeze. But you can always pop into Starbucks and ask for a third of a cup of boiling water into which you put the bottle to warm. If you're not in civilisation, you can buy travel bottle warmers, flasks and all sorts of equipment for keeping bottles cold, warm, or just right.

Combining breast and bottle

If you give formula too early, you can scupper breastfeeding because it can mess up your developing 'supply and demand' system. So if you're worried your baby isn't getting enough milk, always try other things first *(see page 105)*.

Once breastfeeding is established, however, the odd bottle can come in handy and your milk supply will quickly adjust to not giving a certain feed if you do it regularly (many parents give a bottle last thing at night, believing this helps the baby sleep longer – though there is no actual evidence that this is the case). You should be able to keep breastfeeding for the other feeds if you do this, but it's worth knowing that it might lower your milk supply more than you'd want. As a one-off – say if you want a night out – a bottle of expressed milk or formula can be very useful, though you may return home looking like you've had a boob job. If you leave your breasts full you could develop mastitis, so either take your pump with you and sneak off to pump at 'feed time' or, when you get home, pump fully if your baby does not need a feed.

How to switch from breast to bottle

- You don't *have* to use a bottle: a sippy cup will do.
- Cut one feed at a time – breasts can get engorged or develop mastitis if you stop quickly.
- Start when your baby isn't too tired or starving.
- Get someone else to do it: leave the room entirely so she can't even *smell* your boobs, and let her dad, granny, grandad, aunt or whoever do the first few bottle feeds.
- Persevere: some babies are very resistant to the whole idea and it can take days or even weeks to get used to it.

Starting solids

When babies start eating 'real' food they suddenly seem different: mini people, sitting up at the table with a bit of toast and Marmite of a morning, not babes in arms. But while strangely satisfying, weaning can also be worrying. What should you give your baby? When? How? How much? Here's your basic guide.

When?

Six months old is the official kick-off point, but some babies do seem ready for solids a bit earlier than this. It's a very bad idea to wean before four months: your baby's digestive system just isn't up to the job. But if your baby seems ready before six months, do talk to your health visitor. Babies born prematurely may have different feeding needs, so talk to your GP or health visitor about weaning schedules if your baby was born early.

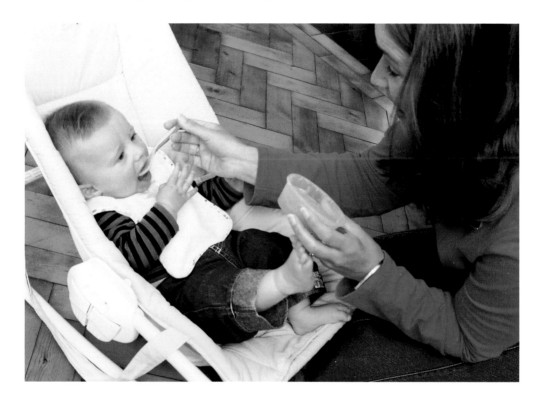

YOUR BABY'S LIKELY TO BE READY IF SHE:

- Is around six months old
- Can sit up (even if supported)
- Is still hungry when she's had a milk feed and you've tried giving her more milk
- Is curious when you're eating and tries to put food into her mouth or seize handfuls from your plate
- Has been sleeping through the night but then starts waking up demanding milk

- Foods that contain gluten (wheat-based food) such as wheat flour, bread, breakfast cereals and rusks
- Nuts and seeds including peanut butter and other nut spreads
- Eggs
- Fish and shellfish
- Citrus fruits, including citrus fruit juices
- Soft and unpasteurised cheeses

All of the above, except nuts and seeds, can be introduced at six months.

How?

From about six months, babies can be propped up in a high chair with cushions so that they can sit unaided. Start at a time when she's neither tired nor starving hungry (a bit hungry, mind, or she'll just think you've invented some weird game) and go at her pace: there's no rule. The overall aim is to get your baby eating 'with the family': that is, enjoying a variety of ordinary foods at roughly three meals a day, with water or milk to drink (in a sippy cup) at each meal and a couple of snacks plus some milk in between.

THE STANDARD WEANING METHOD

The usual advice is to start halfway through a milk feed by offering a teaspoon or so of baby rice mixed with breast milk or formula so that it is about the texture of double cream. Gradually, over a few weeks, you introduce some puréed fruit or veg and other foods at a second then a third mealtime, going at your baby's pace and offering your usual milk feeds in between (your baby will gradually want less milk as she learns to eat more food). Offer some new food every couple of days and give her as much as she wants to eat. The idea, here, is to move from purées to mushed up food then bigger lumps. By the time your baby is on three solid meals a day, you'll probably drop at least one milk feed. Alongside all this you offer 'finger foods' such as carrot sticks or breadsticks, which your baby holds and gnaws on with her surprisingly hard gummy mouth. (Beware: packaged finger foods such as rusks tend to contain sugar and some of the organic baby's first finger food-type products are hardly different, sugar-wise, from bunging her a Mars bar. Always check the labels.)

A FEW WEANING TIPS:

- **Stop when she wants to stop, even if you think she's hardly eaten.**

- **Keep trying: according to Cambridge nutritionist Dr Toni Steer, 'It can take a baby or child several tries to get used to a new food. If she refuses it even half a dozen times, it does not necessarily mean she doesn't like it.'**

- **Encourage self-feeding.**

- **Stay calm: never show her you are wound up by her refusal to eat anything.**

- **Stay nearby when your baby is eating in case she chokes.**

SOME SIMPLE HYGIENE RULES:

- **Wash all feeding equipment thoroughly.**

- **Throw away any food your baby hasn't eaten.**

- **Don't refreeze warmed food if it isn't used.**

- **Wash your hands before preparing food and after you've touched raw meat.**

- **Store raw meat away from other food in the fridge.**

- **Stir any food that's been in the microwave (and check it's cooled before giving it to your baby).**

What?

You want to use normal food (unsalted and unsugared) whenever you can. This doesn't mean you have to be hunched over recipe books at 2am creating organic sweet potato purée. It is fine to serve up your own (salt/sugar-free) lasagne, or some cooked carrots from last night's dinner. Indeed, if your baby is six months plus, you might want to try a simpler approach altogether...

'BABY-LED WEANING'

This weaning 'method' is the increasingly popular brainchild of Gill Rapley, a health visitor for twenty years. Many parents swear by it as the route to hassle-free, non-fussy eating. The basic idea is incredibly simple. At six months a baby is developmentally ready to pick up, chew and swallow real food. Therefore, all you need to do to wean your baby at this stage is to sit her in a high chair, lay out appropriate foods, and let her get on with it.

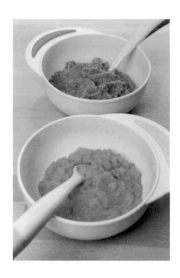

The key with this 'baby led' approach is that you must stop yourself from 'helping' by putting things into your baby's mouth or holding the food for her (though do supervise!). The idea is that she explores food and learns how to feed herself, whilst feeling in control. At first not much food actually goes in, it's mainly about curiosity and exploration so keep milk feeding on demand (milk will be the primary source of nutrition until your baby gets the hang of eating to satisfy her hunger.)

Many parents – usually with their second or third babies – inadvertently end up doing something like 'baby led' weaning. I certainly never touched the blender with Ted, my third baby: I gave him a chunk of something to keep him quiet and quickly realised that he could happily feed himself, so we skipped the purée/mush stage entirely.

If you do decide to wean this way, make sure your baby is six months or older – that is, developmentally ready to sit up and chew. *Baby-led Weaning* by Gill Rapley and Tracey Murkett (Vermilion, 2008) lays out the whole approach very clearly.

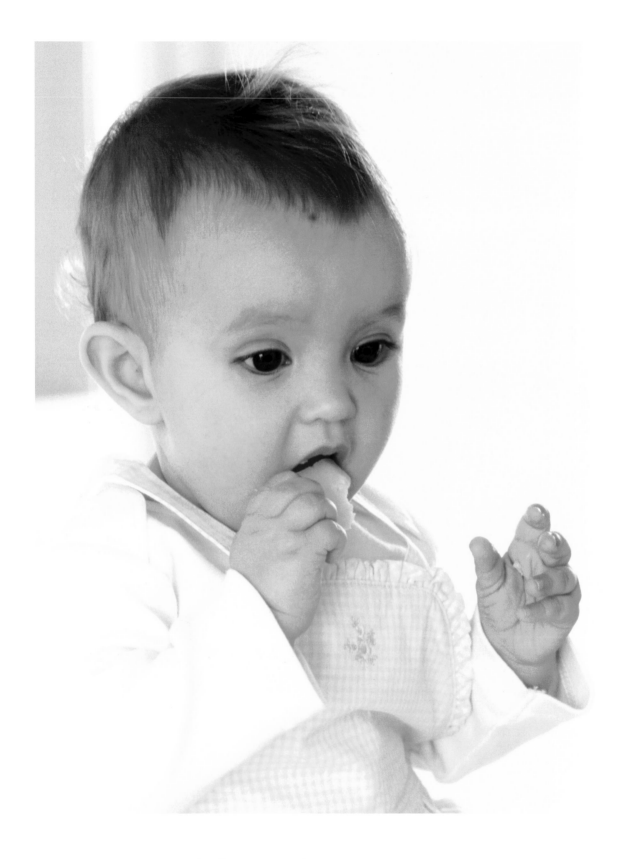

How much milk?

Your baby should carry on having breast milk or about 500–600 ml (about a pint) of formula a day. Though dairy products like cheese are fine to eat, only switch to cow's milk as the main drink when your baby is one (she needs the special nutrients in formula or breast milk). By the time she's eating three good meals a day you should be giving her water in a sippy cup with her meals, and three to four milk feeds (breast or bottle) in between. As she gets bigger she'll want a small snack (fruit, say) with her mid-morning and mid-afternoon milk feeds. Babies and small children need to eat little and often because their tummies are so small.

By the age of nine to twelve months, your baby should be less dependent on milk and should be having a more adult-type diet with three meals a day containing a wide variety of foods, two or three healthy snacks and about a pint of milk.

What not to feed your baby

- Salt. A baby's kidneys can't cope with salt added to cooking (some ingredients, like bacon and cheese, do have some salt in them which is OK in small quantities). Ideally, when cooking family meals, leave out the salt so your baby can eat it too.
- Sugar. Only give things with sugar occasionally as it will encourage a sweet tooth and tooth decay.
- Honey. This can, rarely, contain a type of bacteria that can cause infant botulism. After the age of one, babies are big enough to cope with honey.
- Whole nuts. A baby or small child can easily choke on them *(see also the section on allergies on page 120).*
- Very high-fibre breakfast cereals: they can be hard for babies to digest, so avoid things like All-Bran.
- Low-fat or fat-free products: babies need the calories from full-fat foods. Adult healthy-eating guidelines do not apply to babies: they have quite different nutritional needs. Your baby should have full-fat products until she's two years old, when she can have semi-skimmed.
- Processed foods such as crisps and biscuits. They're nutritionally useless.

Allergies

Your baby is more likely to develop allergies if you've got a family history of eczema, asthma or hay fever. But even if your family is non-allergic, it helps to introduce new foods one at a time so that if something flares up you can isolate the culprit. The main foods to watch are peanuts and those containing gluten.

If you or someone in your family is allergic to peanuts, talk to your health visitor or GP and don't give peanuts to your child until she is at least three years old. If there is no peanut allergy in the immediate family, you can give your baby peanut products from six months, but don't give her whole peanuts or other whole nuts until she's much bigger because she may choke – aged five is the official advice.

'Beware of becoming allergy-obsessed. Even if you've decided bread makes you bloated, don't impose this on your baby.'

If you or someone in your family is genuinely allergic to gluten, talk to your GP before you give your baby any wheat-, rye- or barley-based foods. The Coeliac Society has more information (see **Contacts**).

Finally, beware of becoming allergy-obsessed. Even if you've decided bread makes you bloated, don't impose this on your baby. Babies need a wide variety of nutritious foods, so always talk to your GP before cutting anything out.

What is a balanced diet?

ULTIMATELY YOU'RE AIMING FOR SOMETHING LIKE THIS EVERY DAY:

- Lots (two to three servings) of starchy foods like potatoes, rice, wholemeal bread and unsweetened breakfast cereals
- Lots (include some in most meals where possible) of fruits and vegetables
- A fair bit (one or two servings) of protein: soft cooked meat, fish, egg, tofu or pulses
- A pretty small amount of fat (butter, cheese, mayo), oils and sugary food

Three healthy eating ideas

1 | Porridge is a quick, nutritious breakfast – make it with whole milk and put a bit of banana in if you like, but avoid honey or sugar.
2 | Red meat (beef, lamb and pork) is an excellent source of iron – simple mince cooked with a tin of tomatoes and some peas makes a good baby-friendly meal. A batch of lentils with veggies chopped into it is also really nutritious.
3 | Eggs are a quick, nutritious and cheap source of protein: boiled, mashed and scrambled all work well.

AND THREE MORE

1 | Mashed avocado on toast with sliced peach for pud
2 | Boiled egg and toast soldiers with cherry tomatoes and baby yoghurt for pud
3 | Pitta bread, hummus and grated carrot, with chopped banana and vanilla ice cream for pud

Making it easy on yourself

There's actually no need, mostly, to cook and fuss over separate baby food, even with a smaller baby. When you're cooking for yourself just do a bit extra – of the suitable stuff – and put it in the fridge for your baby's next 'ready meal', or even better give it to your baby to eat with you: family meals can start straight away and are a brilliant way to teach your baby non-fussy, healthy eating. If you do reheat things, make sure they are thoroughly warmed through (then cooled a bit, obviously, so you don't burn your baby's tongue).

SOME USEFUL FOODS

- Cooked veggies or pulses from your own mealtime (cooked with no salt). Give them in chunks to chew on, or mix them into a cheese sauce, or throw them in with some pasta or rice. Bits of cooked broccoli, or carrot slices, or cauliflower bits, are great for little fingers to pick up and munch cold.
- Cooked pasta shapes are fun to pick up and eat.
- Stewed or baked fruits or berries make a great simple pud or a porridge topping.
- Chicken, turkey, ham – with no bones – are great foods for babies to pick up and eat.

Good drinks

When you start to wean your baby, also start to offer her drinks of water alongside the food in a lidded sippy cup. You are aiming to give your baby all her drinks in a cup not a bottle by the time she is twelve to eighteen months old.

- Tap water, formula and breast milk are the best drinks all round (after six months you don't have to boil your tap water).
- Give diluted juice in a sippy cup at mealtimes if you feel the need (about one part juice to ten parts water), but don't give it in a bottle or cup to carry around as this is bad for her teeth.

Bad drinks

- Squashes, fizzy drinks, flavoured milk and juice drinks, or 'diet' drinks of any kind: they are bad for teeth, sweet-tooth inducing and can fill them up so they don't eat properly.
- Tea, coffee or anything caffeinated. For obvious reasons.
- Cow's milk (it doesn't give your baby the right nutrients found in formula or breast milk) until she's one – when it should be full-fat.

Vitamin supplements?

We're all so confused about this sort of thing, but the advice is quite simple.

If you are still exclusively breastfeeding after your baby is six months old, you should give her vitamin drops containing vitamins A, C and D. Ask your health visitor for advice on which kind to get.

If your baby is bottle-fed and/or is drinking 500 ml (about a pint) of formula a day, you don't need to do this because formula is fortified with vitamins already.

Veggie babies

It's fine to have a vegetarian (or even vegan) baby, but you need to be sure she's getting protein from a mixture of foods, and enough iron.

The Vegetarian Society has an information leaflet about feeding babies and children, and the British Nutrition Foundation is another good source of advice and ideas for feeding babies and children (see **Contacts**).

GOOD IRON-RICH FOODS ARE:

- Well-cooked eggs
- Pulses
- Cooked and puréed dried apricots
- Green vegetables

Five keys to weaning success

1 | Buy bibs. Lots of them.

2 | Be blasé. In your weak, desperate moments, remember this: no healthy child will starve herself. The key to weaning (and indeed feeding your small child generally) is the exact opposite of everything you've learned elsewhere in this book. It's simple: never show you care. A small baby will pick up on your anxiety about her eating. Bigger babies (and children) will even learn that – at last! – they have power. Pretend to be completely blasé about what your baby eats even if you have to go into a padded room and scream for ten minutes after each attempted mealtime. Do not fret, get cross or cajole: just breezily remove the dinner if, after ten or fifteen minutes, you are getting nowhere. Get down from the table. Try again later.

3 | Make it normal. Put your baby in the high chair at the table and eat meals together when feasible. And model great eating habits ('Carrots! Broccoli! Yummy!'). This, any nutritionist will tell you, is your best hope of fostering a healthy relationship with food.

4 | Accept fickle feeding. Your baby's enjoyment of any meal will, almost invariably, be in inverse proportion to the amount of time you spent creating it (well, up to a point: try slaving over chocolate chip cookies if you want to see gratitude ...) She may also wolf down a vast bowl of roasted veggies one day and reject them in disgust the next. See 'Be blasé' above.

5 | Limit sweets. Don't go mad even on healthy sweet stuff like bananas, pears or plums. Babies naturally have a sweet tooth and if you stuff her with sweet fruit in the early days, you're likely to find it hard to get her to accept more savoury food like broccoli or green beans. There's no need to avoid anything sweet entirely, but I'd press on with the vegetable medleys, even when you know a banana would disappear in seconds.

Being sensible

OK, I've banged on a lot in this chapter about healthy eating, balanced meals and the avoidance of too many sweets and crappy foods. This is, obviously, the crucial message to absorb. You want your baby to be well-nourished and healthy, not vitamin-deprived, obese, riddled with tooth decay or potentially ill because you have fed her inappropriate foods. But – and it's a big but – *try not to get obsessed by it all.*

A good friend of mine, a mother of five, recently held a barbecue. One woman brought along her ten-month-old baby. There was good-quality, delicious food everywhere – much of it entirely suitable for a ten-month-old baby to sit and chomp. The woman, however, spent most of the barbecue in the kitchen puréeing organic vegetables. She – and the baby – both had a miserable time (Mummy frazzled and cut off from social contact, baby hungry and frustrated, surrounded by food). If you catch yourself doing this sort of thing, try to take a step back. Babies are human. They are designed to eat real food. A ten-month-old (indeed, even a six-month-old) can be given a well-cooked and cooled corn on the cob to gnaw, or a bread roll to munch, or batons of cucumber, or any number of 'normal' foods (as long as the adults keep an eye on her to make sure she doesn't choke or grab anything hot or otherwise ill-advised).

If you're puréeing your nearly one-year-old's meals – unless there's a good medical reason to do so – stop. You're aiming to have a happy, non-fussy, self-feeding baby who eats like a regular human being. This is not the way to do it.

Many of us these days are obsessed to the point of craziness about how our babies eat. So here are some dos and don'ts that may help you to keep things in perspective, and encourage your child to eat in a normal, balanced way.

DO:

- Follow the basic guidelines laid out in this chapter.
- Stay relaxed: part of teaching your baby to eat healthily is teaching her to enjoy a lovely variety of foods – some savoury, a few sweet, some healthier than others – in a relaxed and low-key way.
- Use your common sense: no, your baby shouldn't have too much salt (don't add it habitually to your cooking or give her high-salt foods); but it's fine for her to eat things like shop-bought bread, or cheese, that may contain small amounts of salt.
- Let her feed herself as soon as she's interested. You want her to feel in control and confident about eating. Sitting pinned to a chair while

mummy and daddy spoon goo into your mouth is neither an empowering nor a sensible longer-term eating strategy.

- Occasionally let your baby have a treat. Obviously keep this under control, but it's fine to make an apple crumble once in a while, let your baby enjoy a chocolate pudding, or a biscuit from time to time. This is normal eating. My son went to nursery with one boy who was forbidden sugar of any kind (not for medical or even behavioural reasons). This poor toddler would sit and cry as the others had a biscuit, or poured custard on their stewed fruit. The staff – and I agree with them here – felt it was bordering on child abuse.

DON'T:

- Limit her food intake: let her appetite guide you, even if you think she's eating like a horse, is 'greedy' or 'chubby' (talk to your doctor or health visitor if you have genuine concerns about her weight, but don't act independently).
- Decide without medical advice that your infant has 'food allergies' and start cutting out food groups. Follow the guidelines, and if you are at all concerned about her reaction to certain foods, see your GP.
- Impose your own food anxieties and hang-ups on your baby. Keep a sense of balance if you possibly can, even if eating is fraught for you. Ask your health visitor or GP if you really don't know whether some food or behaviour is OK or 'normal'.

Many of us relax the rules considerably with subsequent babies. My first baby didn't taste chocolate until her first birthday. My third was certainly familiar with it from much earlier on and is the least fussy eater of my three – probably because I let him get on with it. I was so much more relaxed (and busy) third time around and couldn't possibly police him in the way I did my first baby. The point is, babies need to be fed like normal people, within certain sensible and healthy limits. You don't want to produce a child so anxious about food that she either won't eat anything at all, or – as she grows up – will binge madly on unhealthy ('forbidden') food whenever she can get her hands on it. It's not easy, but if you find yourself making vegetables into smiley faces at every meal, or panicking when a granny offers your ten-month-old a chocky bicky, try to chill out. You'll be doing your baby – and possibly her future relationship with food – a huge favour.

If you're still anxious, the Food Standards Agency has a good clear website that you may find helpful: www.eatwell.gov.uk/agesandstages/.

Yes, yes, but how are *you* eating?

It's all very well feeding your child balanced, nutritious meals involving many carrot sticks, but what about you? Most of us are so obsessed with pumping our babies full of nutrients that we completely forget about our own meals and eat a load of rubbish.

'Do you feel fat? Of course you do. You just had a baby. You've achieved a miraculous feat and the resulting size of your knickers is, or should be, irrelevant.'

SIX EASY WAYS TO EAT MORE HEALTHILY:

1 | Make your own 'ready meals' – make soup or stews in large batches and freeze them. These will be cheaper, healthier and less lardy than the ready meals you buy in the shops. Freeze them in individual portions so you can defrost them quickly.

2 | Make it easy to lay your hands on energy-giving, not energy-draining, snacks: fruit, dried fruit, nuts, wholemeal toast, wholemeal hot cross buns. Rid your cupboards of crisps, choccies and bickies, which will give you bursts of energy then sugar crashes (when you feel drained and crave more sugar).

3 | Snack on some of those carrots sticks yourself: snacking on raw veggies will bring you closer to having your 'daily five' portions of fruit and veg, and may help you cope with the snacka-thon that child-rearing can become.

4 | Sit down and eat meals with your baby when it's appropriate – you can have lunch together at least. This will make you sit down and eat a proper meal rather than Jaffa Cakes throughout the day.

5 | Eat breakfast: this is genuinely a good idea for your blood-sugar levels (studies show people who eat breakfast are actually less likely to be overweight, possibly because they don't kid themselves they haven't eaten, then stuff themselves at other meals). Porridge with fruit is always a good option.

6 | Breastfeeding mothers are advised to take vitamin supplements containing 10 µg vitamin D a day.

Do you feel fat? Of course you do. You just had a baby. You've achieved a miraculous feat and the resulting size of your knickers is, or should be, irrelevant. But of course most of us don't see it this way. However, one thing worth knowing is that it's a *very bad idea to diet if you are breastfeeding*. Loony celebrities who appear skinny and buffed weeks after giving birth are – essentially – starving themselves, having tummy tucks, working out with personal trainers, being fed by chefs and, probably, causing their bodies long-term damage. Nice.

SOME SENSIBLE WEIGHT-LOSS TIPS:

- Don't expect breastfeeding to be your miracle cure. While breast-feeding allegedly uses up calories (up to 600 a day) many of us don't lose any weight while doing it, possibly because we stuff ourselves with comfort food and don't get enough exercise.
- Think healthy not restrictive: pregnancy and breastfeeding will deplete your body's natural resources (such as your calcium supply) if you don't have adequate nutrition. If you focus on healthy eating you are likely to lose a bit of weight simply because you will not be eating pizza at every meal. *(See above for some ideas)*.
- Put away your bathroom scales. Only get them out some time after your baby's first birthday. Use your clothing as a less fraught measure of where you are on the baby-fat scale.
- Get some exercise when your doctor OK's it *(see page 63)*.

The first year is not the time to beat yourself up about your inability to squeeze into your pre-pregnancy jeans. Being the mother of a pre-verbal child is, in my opinion, a fabulous excuse for having a tummy that drapes over your waistband. And when your baby is too big to provide this excuse? That's what magic knickers are for. Or second pregnancies ...

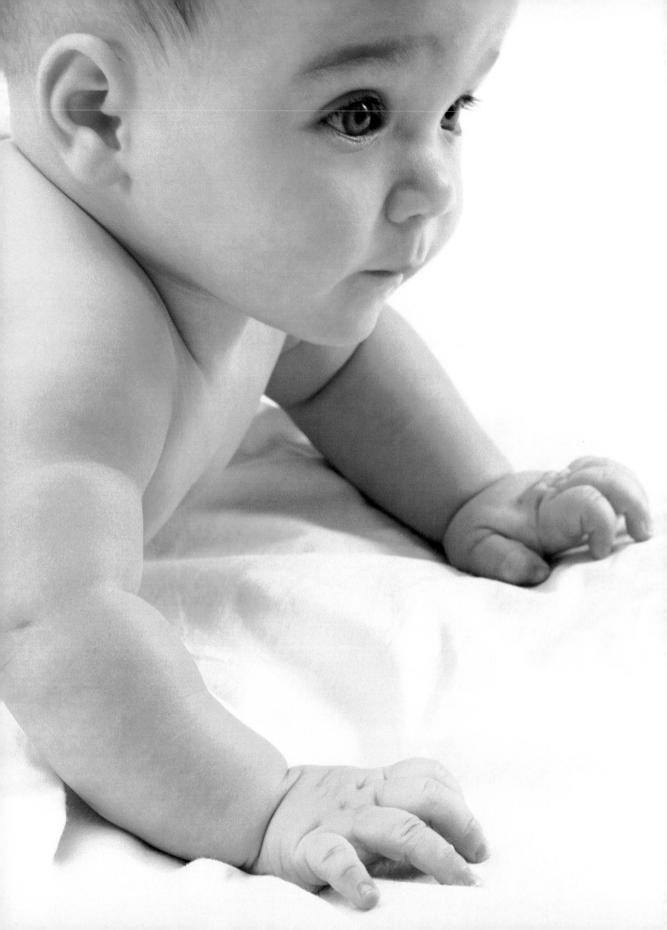

grow

How your baby grows and develops in the first year

We're all obsessed with how 'well' our babies are growing and developing. While it's important (and fascinating too) to make sure your baby is growing healthily, it's also important – for most of us – to take a chill pill from time to time on this one. Babies grow and develop at different rates and most worries we have turn out to be groundless. So, as you pore over this chapter to find out what your baby 'should' be doing at any given time, try to keep an eye on the big picture too. It'll save you a whole lot of first-year angst.

How it happens in the first twelve months

Obsessing on your baby's growth statistics and furtively comparing his developmental progress to that of other babies is entirely futile. But we all do it. The truth is that babies grow at their own pace. Boys are, on average, heavier and taller than girls, and grow at a different rate; Caucasian babies are, on average, larger than babies of Asian origin; babies of Afro-Caribbean origin are, on average, larger than Caucasian babies. Breastfed babies gain weight at a different rate to bottle-fed babies. Twins, multiples or premature babies may stay small in relation to other babies for a long time.

What matters is that your baby is growing healthily – for him. As for the developmental milestones we're all obsessed by, all I can say is beware the mother-in-law ('Is there something wrong with him? Mine were all playing table tennis at six months!') and allow your own mother great poetic licence ('But I had you all out of nappies by your first birthday!').

When your baby is a few days old you will be given a little book in which your child's development and check-ups are recorded. When your baby is born, his weight, length and head circumference are usually recorded in this book. He is then monitored at certain points over the next few years by the health visitor to check that he's growing healthily. There are two official developmental checks in the first year (at six to eight weeks then at eight to nine months), and the health visitor should send you an appointment for these. These check-ups, as well as recording your baby's growth, are about general well-being – how you're coping – so use this time to talk through any parenting issues and worries you have.

THIS IS ROUGHLY HOW A BABY PUTS ON WEIGHT:

- **In the first few days he may lose about ten per cent of his body weight.**

- **By about day ten he's likely to have gained this back.**

- **After this, weight gain is usually about 2 lb a month (just under a kilo). This can, however, go in fits and starts.**

- **In the next six months, weight gain slows up (to about 1 lb (½ kilo) a month).**

- **Most babies double their birth weight by about four or five months and treble it by a year.**

Weight

Most new mothers become paranoid about their baby's weight gain. But what actually matters is your baby's general health, well-being and growth *over some weeks*, rather than the week-by-week ounces and pounds. So unless there's a good reason to do so, I would avoid showing up at the baby clinic purely for weekly weigh-ins – it's likely to make you pointlessly anxious.

LITTLE FATTIES

Some babies are naturally really chubby – think Sistine Chapel cherubs – and unless you're stuffing them with cakes and crisps, most of the chub gradually dissipates, often when they start crawling or walking. Don't limit your baby's healthy food if you think he's 'too fat' (but equally, don't insist on him finishing every feed). As the Child Growth Foundation spokesman puts it, 'Healthy babies don't starve or overfeed themselves.'

Height

Most babies grow on average 25-30 cm (10-12 in) in the first year, and their head becomes more in proportion to their body (newborn babies actually have gargantuan heads compared with their bodies when you think about it). Again, height increases aren't always steady.

Sight

Your newborn can see clearly at a distance of 20-25 cm (8-10 in). This is roughly where your face is when you breastfeed. Isn't nature clever? He will initially see contrast better than colours, which is why those black and white baby mobiles are so exciting for him.

At six weeks his eyes will be able to focus further and will both start to work together. By three months he'll see colours well. By six months he can see more detail, and by twelve months he should be pretty much seeing everything.

Black and white objects are thrilling for your new baby (he sees contrast better than colour).

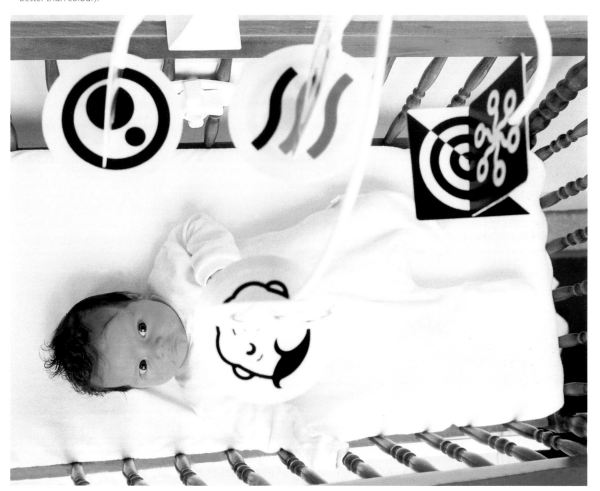

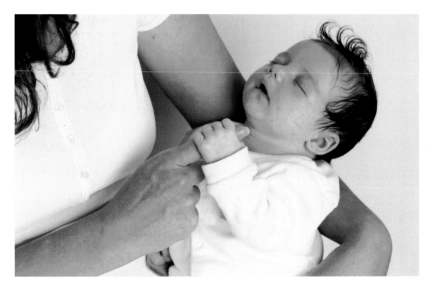

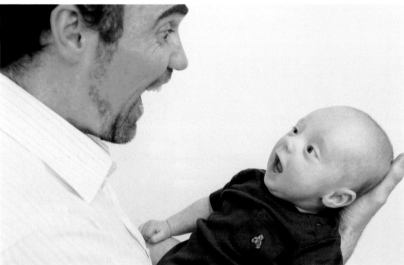

At birth, your baby will grasp your finger *(top)*, and even mimic your daft expression *(bottom)*.

Hearing

At birth he'll recognise his parents' voices, will turn his head when he hears you and should startle at a loud noise. Most newborns have a hearing test before they leave hospital. Their hearing will be checked at the six to eight week check-up and eight to nine month check-up.

Touch, taste and smell

Babies don't just touch with their hands – they use their mouths too. This is their way of finding out about the world. Imagine what an aubergine would look, smell and feel like to you if you'd never seen one. My god! What is it? Is it alive? It's smooth. Ooooo! It's cold.

It smells funny, grassy, watery. What does it taste like? The everyday world is pretty mind-blowing to a baby.

Newborns can taste just as you can, but prefer sweet things like breast milk. They will recognise their parents' smell (studies show that if a new baby is put between a handkerchief with the mother's smell and one smelling of a stranger, they'll turn towards the mother's handkerchief).

Sugar and spice? Puppy dog tails?

Boys and girls really are different (though we're not talking slugs and snails here). *On average* girls walk sooner, grow faster and at a more regular rate, are more sociable, more interested in people than things and cope better with stress than boys do.

A quick guide to how babies grow

At birth

PHYSICAL

He may be able to 'mimic' you: stick your tongue out and he'll try to do the same. He'll also grasp your finger, turn his head, 'startle' if he hears a loud noise and move his legs in a 'walking' way if held up (*see page 31*). He'll love to be touched, held and cuddled.

LANGUAGE AND UNDERSTANDING

His cries, for different reasons, will sound different (you'll gradually get to know them but you'll almost certainly instinctively react urgently to his pain- or fear-type cries from day one). He'll be very interested in voices and smells and is programmed from birth to be fascinated by faces.

Birth to three months

PHYSICAL

It's all about gaining head control and gradually 'uncurling' his body. By six weeks he'll probably be able to follow a brightly coloured moving toy held about 18-20 cm (7–8 in) from his face. He'll learn to lift his head up while lying on his front, and will kick around if lying on his back. Around six weeks he will begin to discover his hands as 'playthings'. Somewhere around twelve weeks many babies learn to roll over from back to side.

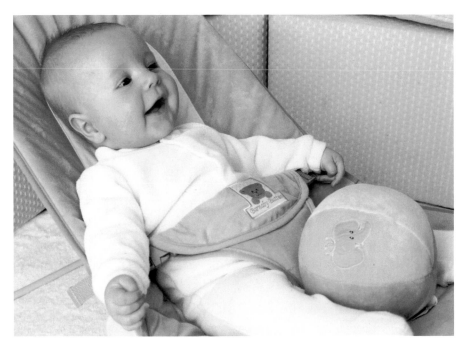

Some time between birth and three months your baby will probably learn to smile – it will, of course, make you go totally gooey.

LANGUAGE AND UNDERSTANDING

He'll gradually start to widen his range of noises. Around four to six weeks he'll learn to smile and will often 'reply' if you speak to him then wait for a response.

Three to six months

PHYSICAL

Hand-eye coordination is really starting now: he'll start reaching out for an object. If you pull him up by his arms, gently, he'll be able to control his head by about four months. Around five months he'll be able to hold an object and get it to his mouth (at first he'll be able to grab it, but not let go). And by six months he'll learn to pass the object from hand to hand.

LANGUAGE AND UNDERSTANDING

From about six months, most babies love pinging up and down in a baby bouncer (burning off all that energy and frustration too).

Initially his sounds will be 'cooing', but gradually he'll start saying more consonants (K, P, B, M), 'babbling' and laughing (around three or four months). He will also smile at himself in the mirror. He'll probably be quite interested in strangers around four months, but will become more 'shy' as his memory skills grow and he understands they are, indeed, 'strange'. By six months he'll be making a good range of repetitive noises, 'ma ma' being one. The D sound comes later. Sorry, Dada.

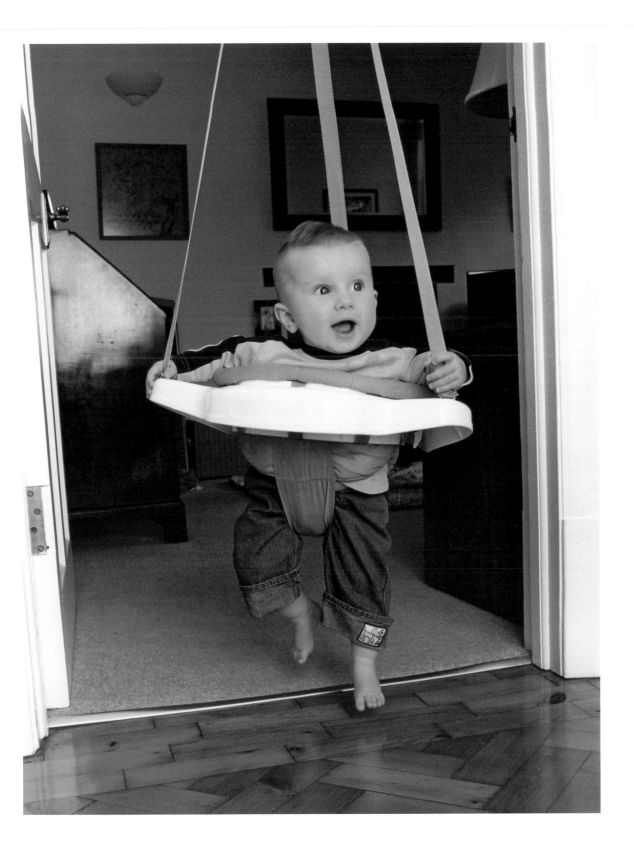

Six to nine months

PHYSICAL

He'll learn to sit up unaided by about nine months – but do put cushions around him while he's learning. He may pull himself up to standing while holding on to furniture, pass things from hand to hand and learn to clap. He might start to feed himself (very messily), and around seven to eight months will learn to pick up smaller objects with his thumb and forefinger. Between six and ten months (often later, sometimes not at all) he may start to crawl – bottom-shuffling, creeping, rocking and going backwards are all normal.

LANGUAGE AND UNDERSTANDING

He'll begin to know his name and will start to imitate your sounds and to understand the word 'no' (at around seven months). He might cry if you leave the room, and may become much more clingy and scared of strangers – this usually happens around eight to nine months). But he'll love other babies, and will reach out to touch them. He'll also get upset when you're angry and will start to learn to 'shout' briefly to get your attention.

Nine to twelve months

PHYSICAL

He'll learn how to let go of an object – give it to you or drop it. Dropping things off the high chair repeatedly will become his favourite game (though possibly not yours). He'll start to wave bye-bye, point at things, hold himself up and maybe 'cruise' round the furniture. Some babies start to take their first steps *(see below)*. He'll be able to build a tower of bricks by the time he's about ten months old, and will probably be able to feed himself finger foods by then too. By the age of one he'll be able to pick up a small object between finger and thumb (a 'pincer' grip).

LANGUAGE AND UNDERSTANDING

He'll be chattering away (not in recognisable words, usually), and by his first birthday he should be able to kiss, understand simple instructions – 'Give the knife to Mummy!' – and say a word or two with meaning.

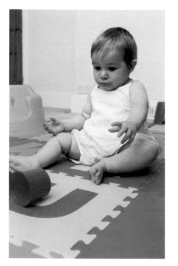

From about six months your baby will learn to sit up unaided.

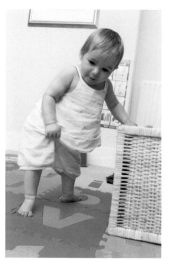

Between nine and twelve months many babies discover how to 'cruise' around the furniture.

Walking

Some babies leap to their feet and waddle off as early as ten months. Others are still happily seated several months after their first birthday. Walking your baby around, suspended by your hands, will not make him walk earlier. Never buy a 'baby walker' (a toy they push to help them 'learn' to walk): they don't teach babies to walk and they do cause an enormous number of accidents every year. Waddling, bow legs, knock-knees, pigeon toes or lurching around with toes out are all completely normal gaits. But if you're at all worried by your baby's gait, feet or legs, mention it to the health visitor.

Looking after your baby's feet

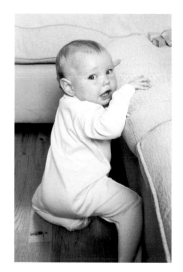

- Keep toenails short – cut them straight across so they don't get ingrown.
- The bones in the toes are soft at birth so you have to be careful not to cramp them – even tight socks and too-small booties can do this. Keep his feet free as much as you can. If the feet of the Babygro get too small, cut them off and use socks at night.
- Only put your baby in proper shoes when he can walk alone. Before this, socks or soft booties are really all you need (get rid of them as soon as he grows out of them).
- Only put his shoes on when he's walking outside – it's better to be shoeless as much as possible.
- Buy shoes made of natural material (leather, cotton, canvas) as it will 'breathe' and isn't rigid.
- Have shoes fitted in a shoe shop that measures them (Clarks is a good place to start), and get his feet measured every six to eight weeks.

Walking safety

Before your baby walks, your house should ideally be 'fall-proof': you may want to shuffle around at walking-baby height and check what he can and can't damage himself on. Then fix it.

See **Chapter Nine** for childproofing tips.

In general, your baby's growth and development is something to revel in, not angst about. During the first year the changes are constant and monumental – more so than at any other time in your child's life, really. You go from suckling a helpless infant to chasing a rampaging, curious, babbling, communicative live wire around in only twelve months. No wonder new parents have those mad, staring eyes. We're totally shell-shocked. In a good way, of course.

Developmental concerns

CHILD-DEVELOPMENT CENTRES

These have teams of professionals (doctors, therapists, health visitors, social workers) specifically to help support children with special needs and their families. Ask your GP or health visitor if there is one near you.

VOLUNTARY ORGANISATIONS

These can be incredibly useful for information and support about specific issues. Ask your healthcare team if they can recommend one.

THE INTERNET

This can be a good place to start, if your problem is not a common one.

SPECIALIST HELP

Your health visitor, GP, social services department or the educational adviser for special needs at your local education department should be able tell you about the specialist services available in your region.

Finding out that your baby has a developmental problem (depending on what it is) can be incredibly worrying and often hard to come to terms with: the baby you thought you had and the one you actually have might be very different. A baby with developmental problems will reach milestones later than average (and sometimes not at all). The key thing is to get information and support about your child's particular condition. A few places to start are listed along the left of this page.

Benefits

You may also be eligible for a Disability Living Allowance, which you can claim on form DLA1. Call the Benefit Enquiry Line for people with disabilities: Freephone 0800 882 200 (in Northern Ireland 0800 220 674). For more information and help, see **Contacts**.

Your baby's teeth

See **Chapter Nine** for signs of illness.

Most babies are born toothless. They have to grow up through the gums, usually beginning around six months with the two in the front (top and bottom). Some babies teethe earlier than this, some much later. It's not unknown for a baby to have no teeth at all by his first birthday, but most have all these 'milk' teeth by the time they're two and a half. A teething baby may be grumpy, waily and upset for a few days with each tooth that comes through. He may wake frequently in the night, dribble rivers, be snotty, red-cheeked, come up in a rash, get a mild fever and chew anything he can get his hands on. There are twenty baby teeth in there, ten at the top and ten at the bottom. Teething, then, is often quite a big deal.

How to soothe your teething baby

Something that seems like 'just teething' might actually be an illness – bear this in mind while tending the teething. However, if your baby is in discomfort from teething, you could try the following:

- Give him something hard and non-sugary to chew on: a teething ring (you can get ones full of a kind of 'gel' that you put in the fridge – cold is soothing), a breadstick or a peeled carrot straight from the fridge.

- Try sugar-free teething gel (you can buy it in chemists and supermarkets). Rubbed on the gum this can give temporary relief.
- At night, or if he is obviously upset by teething pain, you might want to give baby pain-relief medicine *(see page 162)*.
- Some people swear by homeopathic teething remedies (you can even buy them in Boots).

How to look after your baby's teeth

Avoid prolonged or regular contact with sugary food and drinks. How long the sugary things are in your mouth for is just as important as how many sugary things you eat: sweet drinks (including fruit juice) and lollipops are really, really bad ideas. Keep juice-drinking to mealtimes only, and dilute the juice. Even raisins and dried fruit eaten frequently between meals can damage a baby's teeth.

Start brushing as soon as your baby's teeth start to come through. Buy a baby toothbrush and use it twice a day with a smear of fluoride toothpaste (the organicky-type ones often don't contain fluoride, which is an important ingredient in protecting your baby's teeth). Brushing can be a ridiculous farce at first – baby jaws clamped shut, bashing the brush away. The main thing is to get your baby used to the brushing routine morning and night, so don't get too anal about the whole thing. It'll get easier. NHS dental treatment, by the way, is free for children – so get yours on an NHS waiting list now.

Thumb sucking

Babies do this when tired, bored, frustrated or sleepy. Most thumb-suckers are perfectly happy, and if they give up by the time they are six years old they should have no orthodontic problems at all as a result. For more on sucking, see the section on dummies *(page 94)*.

How your baby grows, develops and learns – whatever challenges you meet – is bound to preoccupy you. And so it should. Most of us are indecently obsessed with our children's development – it's part of loving them. If you can get past the 'shoulds' and the anxiety, and abandon (or at least curb) those knee-jerk, competitive urges, your baby's learning and growth will truly be something to love.

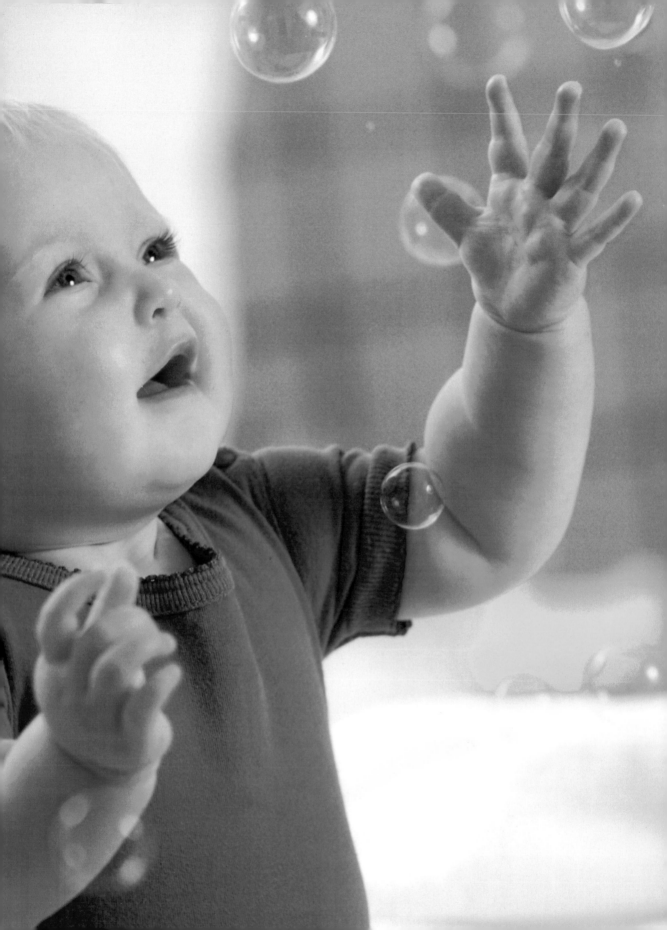

play

Ways to have fun with your baby

What is play? No, no, it's not such a stupid question. These days we're all so busy trying to 'stimulate' our babies, shape them into mini-Einsteins, pre-register them for Sanskrit classes and generally become perfect parents that we forget just to enjoy them. Having fun together is, truly, the best way to 'develop' your baby. And to stay sane. Look on this chapter, then, as a source of ideas for baby fun, rather than instruction in the art of creating an überbabe.

If you forget about being the perfect parent, playing with your baby can be fabulous. 'My biggest surprise is that my son appears to love me back,' says Madeline, mother of Tola, nine months. 'I had not been able to visualise that feeling: when he grins, babbles, giggles – a simple, profound and physical joy.' You'll undoubtedly find it easier to enjoy this sort of thing if you stop worrying about whether you're doing it 'right' or 'enough'.

Your baby does not need to be played with every waking hour because she will learn about the world even when playing alone – with objects, other kids, the dog or simply a pan and spoon on the floor as you cook dinner. Of course, your baby needs plenty of loving interaction: she needs to feel valued and important, and playing with you is a vital and fun part of this communication. But she does not need you, twenty-four hours a day, on your hands and knees showing her flashcards.

'The perfect parent does not exist,' says parenting expert Lorraine Thomas. But a large number of the new parents who come to her for help think it does. 'The stakes for new parents are really high,' she says 'You want to do everything for your child, and you think about all the stuff you should be doing, and you get swamped and overwhelmed.'

Most dads, incidentally, can't wait to play with their babies: they've been at work all day, cooped up with a load of boring old grown-ups, and can't wait to spend their time blowing raspberries into a fat baby's tummy. Maybe it's also because they don't have the same pressures as mums, with all those hothousing baby activities to choose from and hours of the day to fill. They just have a laugh with the baby. In general, playing with the baby is something dads do naturally, and well. Hooray.

How to 'stimulate' your baby

The fear that our babies will go 'unstimulated' has done wonders for sales of ludicrously expensive 'toy' and 'learning' products. Your baby will, in fact, be 'stimulated' by *life*. Take her to the park and she'll feel madly stimulated by the clouds, the sound of a dog barking, the kids on the swings or the smell of cut grass. Babies are immensely easy to stimulate. In fact, small babies quickly get over-stimulated. If you pay close attention to your baby, you'll learn to spot this (fretfulness, loud crying, jerky limbs). There are, however, two things above all that really are worth doing: talk to and read to your baby a lot.

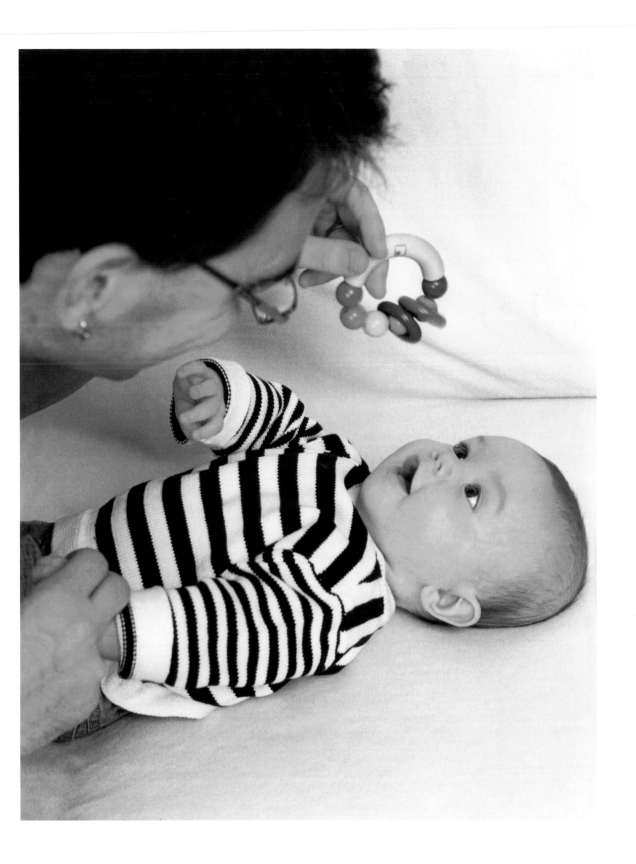

Talk to your baby

Babies – even newborns – respond positively to voices. Talking to your baby will help her to learn language and to feel connected to you. Babies don't learn speech by themselves, they learn by imitation and two-way conversation. Talking to your baby will probably come naturally to you, but if it doesn't:

- Narrate life to your baby ('Now we're going to the kitchen', 'Now I'm in need of a large gin and tonic'), even if you sound as if you'd not be out of place in a psychiatric ward.
- Ask her questions ('Do you like that?' 'Where's it gone?')
- Repeat words and point things out. Animal noises are the first 'words' many babies learn, so go for it, even if you don't know what the armadillo says.
- Talk in short phrases and with a lighter, sing-song voice – studies show babies find this easier to listen to. Listen to her babbled reply, too.
- Sing nursery rhymes. www.thevirtualvine.com or www.songsforlearning.com are good for ideas. Many libraries also have 'Rhyme Time' sessions for babies, where you all sit on the floor and sing rhymes with actions and noises (ninety per cent of library authorities do something like this) .
- Make lots of sounds as you play (like going 'brmm, brmm' with the toy car). Your baby will hear different speech sounds and learn that listening to voices is fun.
- Let your baby 'talk' back: it's amazing how even a very small baby will become quite conversational if you let her get a word in edgeways. Answer her, too, when she tells you something.
- Don't become deranged about all this: sometimes companionable silence is lovely too (something mad mummies often discover with their second babies when they take their foot off the gas a bit).

Read to your baby

Even teeny babies (as young as three months in some cases) can enjoy a good book. The National Literacy Trust, a charity that aims to raise literacy standards, says early book-sharing helps children develop listening, concentration and speaking skills. But above all it's fun. Go for very short books with big bright pictures. Let your baby chew, bash and touch the book. Most babies like looking at pictures of other babies. Animal noises, rhymes and actions are all great. And books that do stuff like rattle or pop up never cease to please. Even a twelve-week-old baby can enjoy a book that squeaks.

For more ideas and inspiration, contact the National Literacy Trust (for details see **Contacts**).

SOME GOOD BOOKS FOR STARTERS ARE:

Where is Maisy's Panda? by Lucy Cousins (Walker Books)
Peek-A-Boo! by Jan Ormerod (Bodley Head Children's Books)

But any touch-and-feel-type books, big 'lift the flap' books or books that make noises are worth a go. Join your local library today. It'll save you a fortune.

Bookstart is a scheme that aims to give all babies in the UK a gift pack including free books and guidance materials – see www.bookstart.org.uk. They also have a regularly updated list of excellent baby books – a fantastic source of ideas.

Good games for different ages

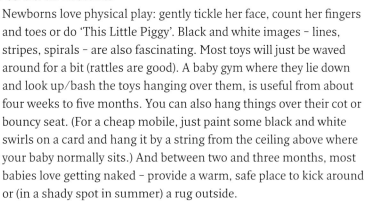

One to three months

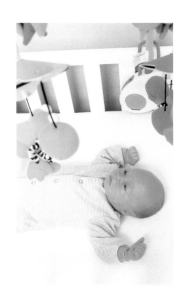

Newborns love physical play: gently tickle her face, count her fingers and toes or do 'This Little Piggy'. Black and white images – lines, stripes, spirals – are also fascinating. Most toys will just be waved around for a bit (rattles are good). A baby gym where they lie down and look up/bash the toys hanging over them, is useful from about four weeks to five months. You can also hang things over their cot or bouncy seat. (For a cheap mobile, just paint some black and white swirls on a card and hang it by a string from the ceiling above where your baby normally sits.) And between two and three months, most babies love getting naked – provide a warm, safe place to kick around or (in a shady spot in summer) a rug outside.

Babies are born with an interest in the sound of voices (particularly yours). Musical/verbal games, nursery rhymes, sing-songs and chatter are all great. Things that make noises are also interesting as your baby gets bigger: try scrumpling a big ball of tissue paper, rattles and big bells. Keep an eye on your baby all the time, though – once she starts putting things in her mouth you really have to be aware of choking possibilities *(see page 168)*.

Basically, with little babies, play is anything that involves learning – about their bodies, feelings, senses or the world. Even getting dressed can be great fun, if you make eye-contact, coo, laugh, tickle or whatever. Give your baby time to respond. It can take her a while to mimic you, or grab something, or smile back, or 'answer' you. Go at her pace, and make it your mission to find out what she likes.

Four to six months

Most of the games above (except the black and white things and possibly the baby gym as she gets towards six months) stay fun. Hand-eye coordination is really developing now, so give her lots of *different* things to touch and look at. Make your own rattles with a water bottle full of coloured pasta shapes or big buttons, but put the lid on tight – soon everything will start to go in her mouth.

You are still her best toy: try playing peekaboo with your face, or hiding an object and making it pop out. Keep up the silly noises, face-pulling, rhymes and songs. Faces are still fascinating, so try mirrors and large photos of people she knows.

And, of course, read books together.

Seven to twelve months

As your baby gets older, don't try to boss her around through play. She'll learn best if she's the boss and you just follow her lead. All the games above are still good, but keep giving her toys one at a time – until she's eight or nine months old she'll be overwhelmed by more than a couple of toys at once.

Around this time she will also be discovering cause and effect, so try toys that do something in response to her actions (like a jack in the box or a toy that plays music when bashed). Things that move (balls, wheeled toys, things that roll) and bashing toys generally (a drum or a pan and wooden spoon) are good, as are simple musical instruments like a tambourine, xylophone or whistle. Pop-up and lift the flap books really come into their own now (they also teach her the concepts of 'in' 'out' 'up' and 'down').

'Real toys are heaven to a bigger baby: most will ditch their toys the minute they think they can get their hands on your iPod or something equally expensive'

Around eight months she may copy you if you scribble with a crayon (give her one too), and might begin to like 'pretend' games such as pretending to eat something. Give her a block, take one yourself, 'Let's have a picnic. Yummy!' You'll be surprised how early babies catch on to make-believe games.

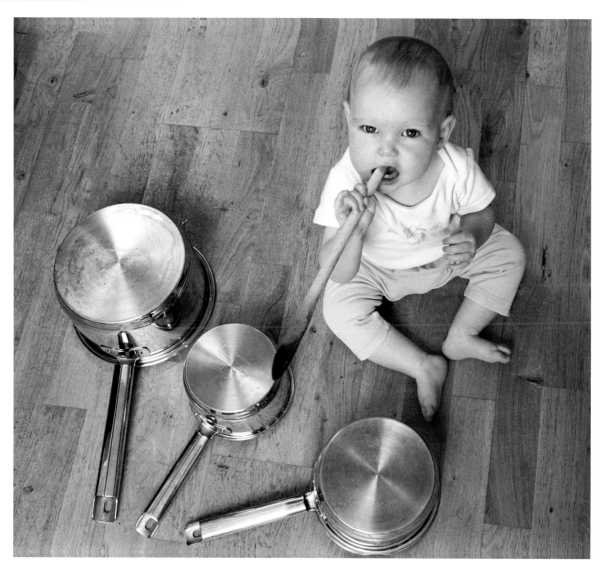

Most babies find household objects infinitely more fascinating than 'proper' toys.

Her manual dexterity will also be improving: building a tower of blocks (and knocking it down), putting things into a box and taking them out again (give her a shoe box and some smallish blocks to put in and out of it). 'Real' toys are heaven to a bigger baby: most will ditch their toys the minute they think they can get their hands on your iPod or something equally expensive and breakable. Instead of pursuing her shouting 'No! No!', give her safe 'real' things to play with like a colander, an old phone or an old tape-player. Finally, there's nothing like a large cardboard box to keep a bigger baby rapturously busy.

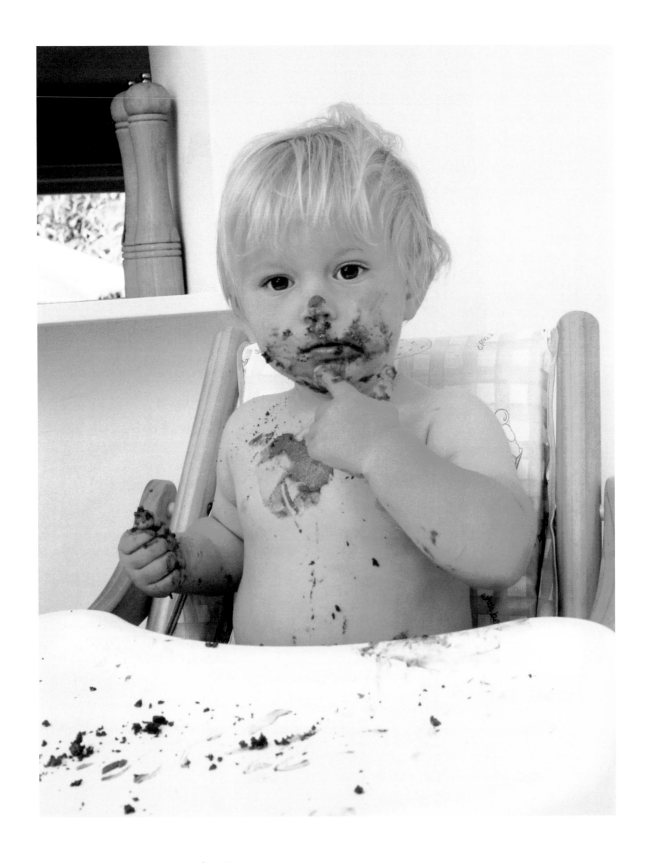

Six basic ways to 'play'

You'll notice these involve neither flashcards, developmental toys, baby Einstein products nor third parties. Just you and your baby, hanging out.

1 | Just let her explore the front room, garden or your face/hands/body if she can't crawl or move around yet.
2 | Cuddle and tickle – it's what most parents are programmed to do (rather than, say, spending six hours a day looking at developmental DVDs).
3 | Be really silly: sing songs, talk nonsense, make silly noises.
4 | Get filthy – parents, particularly mothers, spend so much time clearing up that it can be hugely liberating to get completely filthy. Cover anything expensive and sit back while your baby explores chocolate pudding with her bare hands. On a summer's day let her crawl naked in the garden and get covered in muck, or do a painting with her belly or feet, or play with a bucket of soapy water and some containers.
5 | Dance. Studies show we automatically boogie a bit as we sing to our babies, thereby 'teaching' them rhythm. Babies love to boogie.
6 | Show her how to do things. Towards the end of the first year, it's amazing what she'll be able to learn – pulling off her socks, scribbling, pulling off a big T-shirt. This will be a lot of fun for her (never expect her to do it 'right').

Obviously, this list is potentially endless: just do things you both like doing. My one-year-old and I are, currently, at our happiest 'playing' in Starbucks (he pulls the place apart, I eat the chocolate).

Play it safe

Household objects are truly your baby's best toys, so go easy in Toys 'R' Us. However, do make sure the things you hand your baby are safe. A split yoghurt pot can be sharp, a pan may be heavy if dropped on a small foot. Try to think things through before you hand them over, and remember that everything is likely to be sucked and chewed and dismantled. Avoid anything with small constituent parts – even if you think your baby is unlikely to take it apart. You'd be amazed at the destructive skill of a small baby.

Get filthy once in a while *(left)* – all that tidying up can really get to you ...

Bigger babies and discipline

As you watch your tiny newborn flutter her long eyelashes, it's hard to imagine she'll ever need anything as vulgar as discipline. However, before you know it she will be a toddler. If you don't want her ransacking the house, chewing through electric flexes and generally behaving like a demon, you are going to have to find ways to teach her what's acceptable and safe and what's not. This is, in a sense, a vital part of play.

'As you watch your tiny newborn flutter her long eyelashes, it's hard to imagine she'll ever need anything as vulgar as discipline.'

A FEW TIPS FOR TODDLERS-TO-BE:

- Encourage good behaviour. Praise her when she is gentle and strokes the cat rather than yanking his fur off.
- Be patient. Your baby is not being 'naughty' – in fact, she really doesn't know what 'naughty' is (she's trying to work this out, along with everything else). Help her to learn, gently, what's acceptable and safe and what's not, and do not expect her to remember anything until it's been repeated many, many times.
- Be firm and consistent. If you laugh when she cheekily sticks her finger in the DVD player one day, she'll be confused by your yelling when she posts her toast in the next.
- Frame things positively. Instead of barking 'No! No!' round the clock, *suggest the behaviour you want to see*. When, for instance, she bashes your face, stop her hand and say 'Gentle!', then show her what gentle means – get her hand and stroke it down your cheek. She'll probably think this is a game, and bash you again, but gradually it will sink in.
- Put yourself in her position. It's easy to get annoyed with a rampaging baby, but if you think of it from her perspective, it often becomes clearer why she's behaving like this.

Smacking

Most experts now believe that smacking isn't a great idea, and I'm going to come off the fence here. I am far from being the perfect mother, and I have a dreadful temper when riled (which, with three kids, is frequent); but while I do occasionally lose it, I don't smack them. My reasoning here is that I am trying to bring them up to be non-violent adults who verbalise their frustration and anger instead of bashing people to make a point. I believe that teaching by example is valid (if hard), and can't see any value in hitting them when I'm trying to tell them never to hit, even when they're too young to understand the concept of hitting. All smacking really teaches a child is that Mummy or Daddy has temporarily lost the plot. The notion that the bigger one automatically wins any given argument is also something I'm not keen for them to learn. In short, most child-development experts agree that there are far, far better ways to elicit the kind of behaviour you want to see.

Biting

IF YOUR BABY SINKS HER FANGS INTO YOU OR ANYONE ELSE:

⊙ **Immediately say 'Ow! That hurts!' (This is likely to be heartfelt – it does!)**

⊙ **Immediately put her down, move away from her, or take her away from the baby/child/ person she has bitten.**

⊙ **Try not to get angry – it's not her fault and she's not being 'bad'.**

⊙ **Pick her up again after a minute or two and carry on as normal.**

Some babies, usually towards the end of their first year, bite other babies and sometimes adults. This can be a sign of frustration – they can't tell you verbally what they want – and also a side-effect of teething (biting just feels good). It's normal, and is not a sign that they're in any way maladjusted or victims of 'bad parenting'. It can, however, make playdates a little tense. Have a biting strategy worked out *(see left)* and use it consistently.

You are – patiently – teaching her that biting hurts other people, which is not an easy concept for a baby to grasp, and that it's no fun, because she gets put down or taken away if she does it. If anyone tells you to bite your baby back, for God's sake don't – you're trying to teach by example, aren't you?

Getting Out

Obviously you may not want to spend your entire life making silly noises and smearing spaghetti around your home. Here are some ideas:

Classes and activities

Classes and baby-specific activities get you out of the house, help you meet other parents and allow you to feel incredibly virtuous because your baby is being 'stimulated' to within an inch of her life. But if baby yoga makes you want to reach for the Prozac, *don't feel you have to go*. Your baby will not be missing out on anything developmentally crucial.

FIVE COMMONLY ENJOYED BABY ACTIVITIES:

1 | Baby yoga. Some of the techniques can help a baby's digestion and sleep, and she'll get to see other babies, which is always fun.
2 | Music groups. From about six months, sitting around with a load of other babies, singing and banging tambourines, is fabulous fun for a baby.
3 | Swimming classes. Usually recommended once your baby is immunised, there may be 'water baby'-type classes at your local pool.
4 | Baby massage. Try your yoga centre or natural-health centre.
5 | Parent and baby groups. Fathers are normally welcomed with open arms, even if most of the coffee-drinkers are female. The National Childbirth Trust (NCT) is the best known of these (www.nctpregnancyandbabycare.com), but your local community centre will probably have one too. Online, www.netmums.co.uk is a good way to plug into your local baby scene.

Another interesting trend is baby signing classes, sometimes with singing, that teach your pre-verbal, hearing baby, as young as six months, to communicate with you using sign language before they can use words. Some of the claims seem a bit inflated, but most parents say it's great fun, and useful too. Try www.babysigners.co.uk.

Parks and playgrounds

Most bigger babies (once they can sit) love a good sandpit or swing. And just being outside on the grass can be liberating for both of you. Take sunscreen and a sun hat in warmer weather, and put her in light, loose clothes that cover her skin as much as possible. Take drinks and snacks for both of you, and a nappy bag – because she'll certainly poo.

The supermarket

IT CAN BE BABY HELL. HERE ARE SOME SURVIVAL TACTICS:

- Strap your baby in the baby seat in a trolley (or put her in a sling if she's light enough) – trying to carry her in your arms and shop simultaneously is futile.
- Always feed her before you leave. If you're caught short, many supermarkets now have mother and baby feeding rooms or a café where you can feed your baby while fortifying yourself with twenty Twixes.

- If she's big enough, give her a time-consuming, hand-held snack when she starts getting twitchy – cheese sticks, breadsticks and rusks are all good. I always forget to bring snacks and end up apologetically paying for various boxes of half-eaten food at the checkout. Nobody has ever arrested me for this.
- Ignore all looks, comments and 'suggestions' as you wheel your howling baby through the checkout. You'll soon be in the car, where you can break down sobbing at the wheel and tell yourself 'never again'.
- Shop online. You know it makes sense.

Travel and holidays

Travelling with babies can be an ordeal – at the very least it'll be some time before you'll watch a whole in-flight movie again. But if you let this stop you, you're going to be housebound for the next four years, so I say just do it. And if you go abroad, remember that your baby needs her own passport.

There are many ways to make flights, even long-haul ones, manageable with babies. You can find some good survival tips at www.babyflying.co.uk, and www.tinyflyers.com may even be able to hook you up with an in-flight 'au pair'.

What to consider when choosing holiday accommodation

- Stairs. You can make a holiday with a crawling baby massively more relaxing if you go to a holiday cottage that has only one level (or provides stair gates).
- Equipment. Lots of holiday houses and hotels provide travel cots and high chairs. Going to an overtly child-welcoming place will make your stay a hundred times more relaxing.
- Swimming pools. There's nothing less relaxing with a mobile baby than a swimming pool that's not fenced off. It means you have to watch your (crawling and beyond) baby every second.
- Distance from civilisation. It helps to have a small shop or two within a few miles as you're always running out of something when you have a baby.

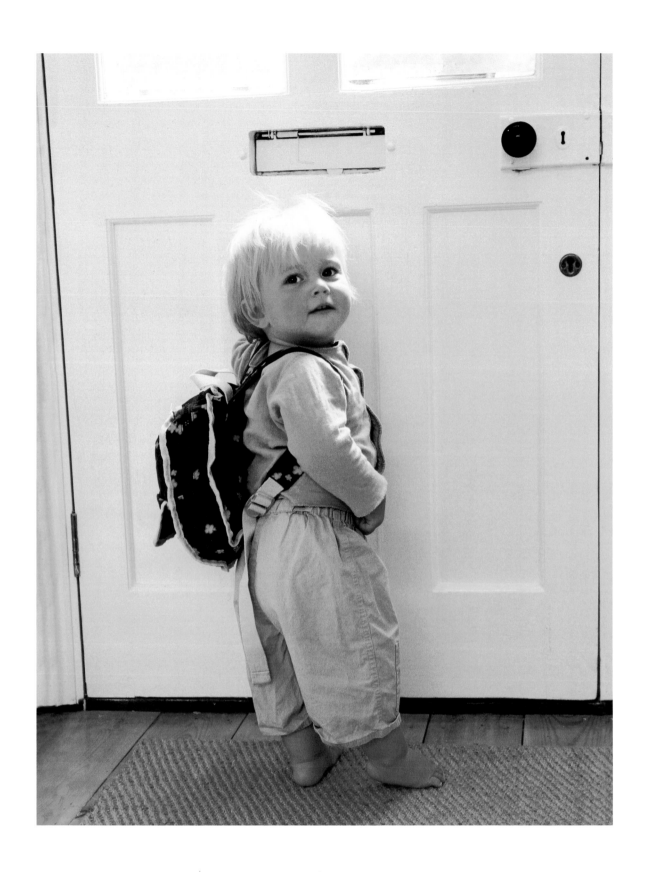

Holiday packing

Try to adopt a spirit of adventure, rather than spend five days trying to recreate 'home' then five days dismantling it all again. The details, of course, will depend on where you're going, but here's a basic list:

- A travel cot (unless you're going somewhere that provides a cot), your baby's Grobag (or other bedding) and any comfort item
- A lightweight travel buggy and possibly a sling if your baby is small
- A car seat, unless you have a hire-car with an infant car seat *suitable for your baby's age and weight*. Double-check this detail with the car-hire company before you leave.
- Food and feeding equipment for the journey and first night
- A rudimentary First Aid kit containing infant paracetamol, insect repellent, insect bite soothing cream or calamine lotion, rehydration sachets suitable for babies in case of diarrhoea or vomiting, small plasters and antiseptic ointment or wipes, and a thermometer
- Weather-appropriate clothing (don't overdo it, you can wash things)
- Sunscreen and sun hat. For babies over six months, always use sunscreen, light protective clothing and sunhats, and keep your baby out of the sun between about 11 a.m. and 3 p.m. For babies younger than six months, try and keep them in the shade wherever possible. For more tips, try Cancer Research's www.sunsmart.org.uk.

WHAT YOU PROBABLY DON'T NEED:

- Two weeks' supply of nappies and wipes. Foreign babies poo too, and unless you are hiking in the outback you will be able to *go to a shop*.
- Your high chair. You can buy handy travel ones that clip on to tables or seats, but you can also just sit your baby on your lap for a week.
- Your steriliser. You can boil or steam things for ten minutes to sterilise them, or take sterilising tablets that you drop into ordinary water.
- Tons of toys. Just take a few (small) favourites and a handful of books.
- Two weeks' supply of baby food. Mostly a trip to the supermarket in whatever country you're visiting will suffice. Just take enough pots to get you through your outward journey.

Flying with babies

I moved to Seattle when my first baby was just over one, and had my second while living there. Frequent transatlantic flights with small children and babies forced me to hone the following survival skills:

IF YOU ARE FLYING ALONE WITH A BABY, THERE ARE A FEW MORE THINGS TO CONSIDER:

- **Ask if your flight is full when checking in – sometimes they will agree to block out the seat next to you if it's not.**

- **Make your carry-on bag a rucksack: most airlines will let you take the pushchair as far as the gates but not on to the plane. You'll need to carry your baby, and all your stuff, on to the plane by yourself.**

- **A baby sling can be useful: then you can push a luggage trolley with two hands.**

- **Be thick-skinned: your baby will cry.**

- Get your baby to suck – breast, bottle or sippy cup – on take-off and landing to stop her ears from hurting.
- Ask cabin crew if you forget something – many airlines keep backup supplies of nappies, baby food and the like. But don't bank on this.
- Book a 'travel cot' or 'bassinette', if the airline has them, for long-haul flights. Ring and check twenty-four hours before you fly that there is one reserved for you, check in early, then shout at people hysterically when they say there isn't one. It can be a battle, but it's worth it.
- Take cheap, new books or small toys. Get them out one by one for novelty value, but don't expect them to entertain your baby for more than about thirty seconds. They're more of a short-term distraction than a way to pass much time.
- Keep your equipment to a minimum (*see below*).
- If you're flying at bedtime, try to give your baby as many normal 'sleep cues' as you can – there's nothing stopping you from putting on her PJs, reading a book, having a bottle, singing that song …
- Be prepared to lose things like socks and toys. You'll stress yourself stupid looking for every tiny thing.
- Get on the plane last. Even though staff encourage you to get on first, it's the last thing you want to do if your baby is at crawling age and beyond. You want her to be zooming round the airport lounge, using up as much energy as possible before you get on.
- If you are travelling as a family, you and your partner may want to get separate seats so one can rest for a bit while the other wrestles with the baby. *Then you swap.*
- Expect to spend about eighty per cent of the flight walking your baby up and down the aisle and the other twenty per cent apologising to everyone around you.

TO DRUG OR NOT TO DRUG?

Some parents will advise you to give your baby an antihistamine or some other mild over-the-counter sedative to help her sleep on a long-haul flight. A word of warning here. I know an anaesthetist who sedated his two small children at the start of a nine-hour transatlantic flight. Both children became hyperactive, so he 'upped' the dose.

They then howled insanely for five hours, crashed out for two, woke up with a 'hangover' and screamed for the remaining two hours. 'Sedatives' can backfire spectacularly.

The best advice I ever got on surviving long-haul travel alone with my two small children was to have a large gin and tonic soon after take-off. This way, you won't care what people think. It works a treat. For more sensible ideas try www.babyflying.co.uk.

WHAT TO PACK FOR LONG FLIGHTS

- Nappy-changing stuff. Think one nappy for every couple of hours of travel time, lots of wipes, travel changing mat, nappy sacks and a couple of muslin squares.
- Bottles/sippy cups
- Cartons or sachets of formula if you are bottle-feeding (bring a couple of extra feeds in case of delays)
- A bottle of water
- Food. Jars of shop-bought baby food are best when travelling. Tupperware containers tend to spill and may need refrigeration. Disposable bibs are fantastic for journeys. And hand-held snacks (ideally ones that take ages to eat, like raisins) are useful for babies who can do finger food.
- A comfort item such as a blankie or teddy
- A cotton sheet or extra blanket to drape over the bassinette and help your baby sleep
- An extra outfit (or more, depending on the length of the flight) for the baby, and an extra T-shirt and sweater for you (your baby will almost certainly throw up and smear food on you)

For more sources of information on travelling with your baby, see **Contacts**.

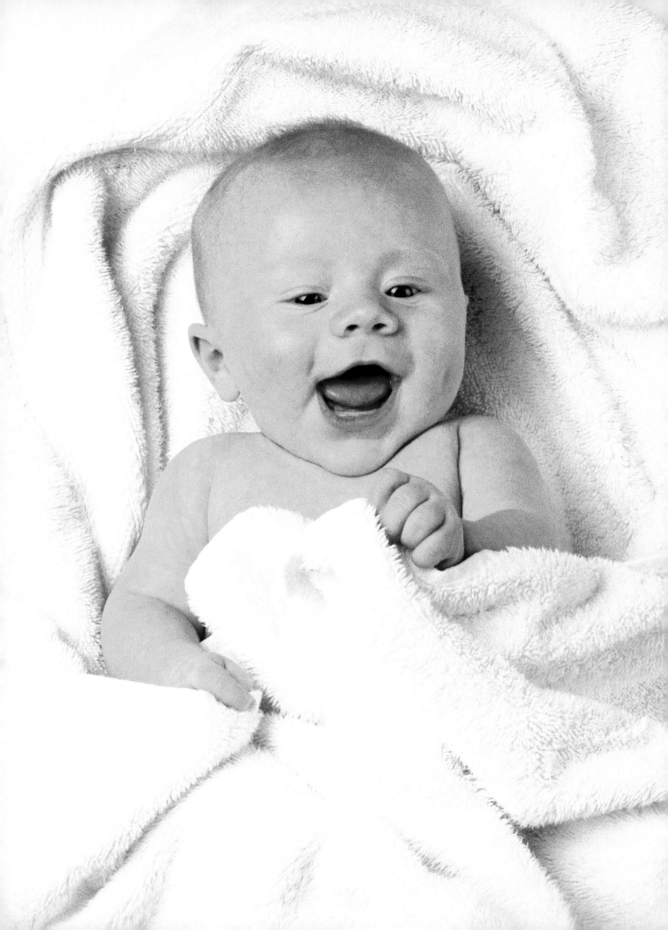

thrive

How to keep your baby safe and well

Keeping your baby healthy and safe is your top priority. A combination of basic information, common sense and instinct will get you a long way. This chapter contains your need-to-know information; the instinct and common sense bits are up to you. But if they've both deserted you, don't panic: your golden rule is if in doubt get help. It's the only way to stay sane.

How to tell if your baby is ill

- You see some sign of illness such as vomiting, a fever, a runny nose or diarrhoea.
- He is behaving oddly or differently. He may be crying a lot, or in a different way or tone, refusing to eat or just looking listless or unusually floppy.
- You just sense or fear he's 'not right'.

It's fine (indeed sensible) to see your GP if you're at all unsure about whether your baby is ill. 'GPs and health visitors are always happy to see or discuss babies,' says GP Louise Hoult. 'We know it can be hard to evaluate babies who aren't well, and that having an ill baby is very tiring, so we tend to be especially sympathetic to new parents.' If you're worried that your baby is sick and you can't get hold of your GP, it's not extreme to take him to the accident and emergency department (A&E) at your nearest hospital. 'It's not up to you to diagnose your baby,' says Dr Liza Keating, a specialist registrar in emergency medicine. 'A&E doctors really do not mind seeing babies. We see them all the time here. We'd much rather see a baby and rule out illness than the other way around.'

When to call an ambulance

YOU SHOULD CALL AN AMBULANCE IF:

- He is unconscious
- He is choking and you can't remove the object
- He is having severe difficulty breathing. Signs include blue lips, struggling to breathe, flaring nostrils, deep indentations of the chest when breathing and inability to finish feeds because he is breathless or sweating when feeding.
- He has had a fit *(see page 162)*. If he seems fine, drive him to A&E; otherwise call an ambulance.
- He is ill and has a purple-red rash anywhere on his body. This could be a sign of meningitis, especially if the rash does not disappear when you press a glass tumbler on it *(see page 165)*.

When to see the doctor
Call the doctor urgently if your baby seems excessively or uncharacteristically fussy or irritable, unusually lethargic or sleepy, is feeding poorly/differently/not at all or is crying in a high-pitched or 'odd' way. If you can't see a doctor urgently, drive him to A&E.

- Has a temperature higher than 37.7°C (100°F) if taken orally that is not responding to infant paracetamol. (Any newborn with a temperature should see a doctor immediately)
- Is vomiting forcefully or more frequently than usual (not just spitting up), possibly with diarrhoea
- Repeatedly refuses feeds for more than six to eight hours
- Has diarrhoea or unusually frequent and watery poos. Moderate diarrhoea is about three loose poos in twelve hours. Severe diarrhoea is about four or more very watery and copious ones in twelve hours.
- Has blood in his poos
- Develops a hoarse cough with noisy breathing
- Shows signs of jaundice – yellowish whites of the eyes and a yellowish or tanned look to the skin *(see page 32 for more on jaundice)*
- Shows signs of dehydration – a dry mouth, dark yellow urine, a sunken fontanel (the soft part on the top of your baby's skull where the bones have not yet joined together), a dry nappy for six to eight hours or fewer than five wet nappies in twenty-four hours once your milk has come in

Prescriptions and NHS dental treatment, by the way, are free while you are pregnant and for twelve months after you have given birth. Your child gets free prescriptions until he's sixteen years old.

Common worries

Temperatures

A fever is a temperature of about 37.7°C (100°F) or over. If taken under the arm, a normal temperature will be about 0.6°C (1°F) lower than if it is taken under the tongue. A normal temperature is anything between about 36°C (96.8°F) and 37°C (98.6°F). As a basic rule, if you rest your forehead on your baby's, it should feel about the same as you (if you're well and haven't just been in the cold or jumping around).

You can buy 'strip-type' thermometers that you hold on your baby's forehead, but they're inaccurate and therefore pretty useless. It can be hard to hold a baby still to take the temperature under the arm. My best anxious-parent investment was a digital thermometer that goes in the ear (like GPs use). It was expensive but is incredibly handy: it takes the temperature in a second and is very accurate. I got it in Boots. Digital thermometers in general are the most accurate.

A little bit of a temperature in itself is not usually something to worry about, but if your baby has a very high temperature or a temperature along with other signs of illness, you should call the doctor *(see above)*. Either way, you want to try and lower his temperature:

- Forget the notion of 'wrapping up' a feverish baby; you want to unwrap him so he cools down. Take his clothes off down to his nappy and keep the room cool (turn down radiators, open a window).
- Give him baby fever medication *(see below)* according to the dosage on the packet.
- If his temperature is still high when you've done all this, try sponging him down (body, arms and legs) with tepid – not cold – water. Lie him on a towel to do this.
- Breastfeed or bottle-feed as normal, but don't worry about solids if he doesn't want to eat.
- Get him to drink frequently – cooled boiled water, milk, watered-down juice.

BABY FEVER MEDICINE

Calpol – infant paracetamol – is a good medicine to bring down a fever, but ask your GP before you give it to a baby under three months old. You can also buy baby ibuprofen, which is safe for babies over 7 kg (15 lbs). If your baby has asthma you should avoid baby ibuprofen unless your GP says it's OK. You should never give aspirin to a child under sixteen years old because it can make them very ill indeed.

Having a 'fit'

There are many reasons why your baby may have a fit, but often it happens with a very high temperature (known as a febrile convulsion): your baby starts sudden jerky, uncontrollable twitching movements, possibly with a frothing mouth and rolling eyes that usually last no more than a minute or two. Though terrifying for you, this is relatively common (three to five per cent of children aged six months to five years suffer from them) and it is hardly ever serious.

If your child has a fit, you need to keep him safe while it's happening. Lie him down (bigger babies can be hard to hold, and you don't want to drop him) and make sure he's not going to bash himself on something or roll off anything. Try and stay calm if you possibly can because he probably needs your comfort most of all. Get someone to drive you to A&E when it's over so doctors can check him over, and do whatever you can to lower his temperature *(see above)*.

If the fit goes on for more than a minute or two, or he has not recovered after thirty minutes (normal behaviour, fully conscious, pupils at their normal size) call an ambulance as he may need more urgent treatment.

Colds

Babies and children can catch a cold eight or more times a year (your baby is building up his immunity to the hundreds of different cold viruses out there). Most colds will get better in five to seven days, and studies show that cold and cough medicines do little to help, so I wouldn't bother with them. Increase the amount of fluid your baby drinks – offer cooled boiled water as well as his usual milk feeds – and put a pillow under the head end of his mattress: it might help him breathe more easily (it tilts him up). Finally, if he has a fever, do what you can to lower it *(see above)*.

Coughs

COUGH TIPS – SEE YOUR DOCTOR IF:

⊙ **The cough continues for more than a couple of weeks. Sometimes persistent coughs can be a sign of asthma.**

⊙ **He also has a temperature and/or breathlessness. This might be a sign of a chest infection.**

⊙ **He's having trouble breathing. If this is the case, see a doctor straight away, even if it's the middle of the night.**

For more information about asthma contact the National Asthma Campaign (see **Contacts** for details).

Coughs often go hand in hand with colds (they are a way for your baby to expel all that mucus). If he is feeding, eating and breathing normally and there is no wheezing, there's no need to worry. Cough mixtures almost certainly are a waste of money. Instead, give your baby frequent warm, clear fluids to drink (cooled boiled water in a bottle or from a spoon for a baby under six months), and offer feeds as normal (which he may decline).

Flu

The symptoms of flu – headache, sore throat, fever, coughing, aches and sometimes vomiting and diarrhoea – can make a small baby very miserable. Usually you'll be able to tell because he'll cry in a different way, will have a fever and will seem obviously unwell. On rare occasions flu can be dangerous for small babies (and children), and some other serious illnesses have flu-like symptoms, so if your baby develops these symptoms, always call the doctor.

Bronchiolitis

This is an inflammation of the respiratory passages in the lungs (bronchioles) that usually affects babies between two and twenty-four months, making them cough, wheeze and breathe quickly or with difficulty. One common virus that causes bronchiolitis is RSV (respiratory syncytial virus). One in twenty children with bronchiolitis have to be taken to hospital to monitor their breathing. This is one reason why, if your baby shows any signs of breathing difficulty, you should always contact the doctor straight away.

Croup

If your baby has a barking, hoarse cough, his breathing is noisy and, when he breathes in, the spaces between his ribs or below his ribcage are sucked inwards, he may have croup. This is an inflammation of the larynx (voice box) and can become serious if it's not treated. Don't panic: croup is very common. But if you can't see the GP within a few hours, take your baby to A&E (you don't need to call an ambulance, just get someone to drive you).

Steam can help temporarily relieve a croupy cough – shut the bathroom door and run the hot tap so the room steams up. Cold and damp air can also help (try opening the window and sitting with your baby by it if it's cold and damp outside). But most of all see a doctor. If it is the middle of the night and you're unsure whether it is croup or not, call NHS DIRECT (0845 46 47) for advice.

Diarrhoea

IF YOUR BABY HAS
DIARRHOEA:

⊙ **Call the doctor if it
continues for more
than twenty-four hours,
or your baby shows any
signs of dehydration,
or is also vomiting or
otherwise seems unwell.**

⊙ **Keep breastfeeding or
bottle-feeding as often
as your baby wants
(offer him lots).**

⊙ **Offer water between
feeds (cooled boiled
water if under
six months).**

Small babies do squitty poos all the time so you might fear you'll never be able to tell if it's diarrhoea or not. But you will: the thing about diarrhoea is that the poos are very, very watery and more frequent than normal. They might smell weird or yukky and be a different colour. Sometimes there may be vomiting too.

Ear infections

A cold can cause an ear infection, usually with a bit of a temperature. Small babies can't always tell where the pain is coming from (or, more to the point, tell *you* where it's coming from), so although a bigger baby may rub or pull at an ear, smaller ones may just seem very unhappy, scream, cry, fuss and wake up a lot.

Ear infections are very common. If you are at all worried your baby may have one, see your GP. Some doctors treat ear infections with antibiotics, others say give Calpol and let it clear up on its own (eighty-five per cent clear up by themselves and many are caused by viruses, which don't respond to antibiotics anyway).

Eczema

One in eight children have a skin condition called 'atopic' eczema (usually if there's a family history of eczema, asthma or hay fever). It often starts when a baby is two to four months old with patches of red, dry, sore skin on his face, behind his ears and in the creases of his neck, knees and elbows. If you notice these symptoms, talk to your GP and contact the National Eczema Society (for details see **Contacts**).

Rashes

Babies often get rashes, and many of them are perfectly harmless. The main rule of thumb is that if you are worried about a rash, or if a rash appears with other illness symptoms such as a fever, call your GP.

Meningitis and septicaemia

Meningitis is an inflammation of the membranes that surround and protect the brain and spinal cord. There are two kinds of meningitis: viral and bacterial. Viral meningitis is generally less serious and most people with it will recover after a few weeks without any specific treatment. Bacterial meningitis, however, can be life-threatening and needs urgent medical attention. One in ten people with bacterial meningitis die.

You can, but do not always, get meningococcal septicaemia (blood poisoning) with bacterial meningitis. This causes a distinctive rash that does not fade under pressure. But you don't always get the rash with bacterial meningitis, so if your baby seems very sick, never wait around to see if a rash appears. He may get some of the following symptoms, not always together, or obviously, or all at once:

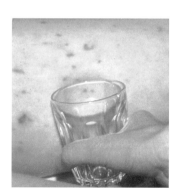

The meningitis rash will not fade when you press a glass on it.

- Fever – sometimes with cold hands and feet
- A high-pitched, moaning cry
- Drowsiness and difficulty waking up
- Refusal to feed or vomiting
- Pale or blotchy skin
- Fretfulness or a dislike of being handled
- A blank or staring expression
- A stiff neck or arched back
- With septicaemia, a rash with red or purple spots anywhere on the body that does not fade when you press a glass on it. The rash can be more difficult to see on black skin so check carefully, especially on the soles of the feet, palms of the hands and inside the eyelids.

The Meningitis Trust has more information – for their details see **Contacts**.

If meningitis is picked up and treated early, the chances of recovery are good. But it is often a big worry for parents (and doctors) as the early symptoms can be the same as those for colds and flu. The main difference with bacterial meningitis or septicaemia is that your baby will usually get very sick very quickly – sometimes within hours. You will almost certainly instinctively know if something is very wrong with your baby. If your baby has any of these symptoms and you feel in your gut that he's very ill, go straight to the A&E department if you can't see your GP immediately. It can also help to call NHS DIRECT (on 0845 46 47), a government nurse-staffed helpline, if you're in any doubt out of GP hours.

Preventing Problems

Immunisations

TWO MONTHS OLD

Polio – dropped on your baby's tongue

Hib (haemophilus influenzae type b) injection

DTP (combined diphtheria, tetanus and whooping cough) injection

THREE AND FOUR MONTHS OLD

Boosters of **Polio, Hib** and **DTP**

THIRTEEN MONTHS OLD

MMR (combined measles, mumps, rubella) injection

In recent years there has been an enormous, media-fuelled hoo-ha about childhood immunisations – particularly MMR. A study, now conclusively discredited, suggested that the MMR could be linked to apparent rising rates of autism and possibly bowel disease. Further studies have not found any link whatsoever. All the evidence is that childhood immunisations are a very good idea – for your baby and the community. (Measles, for instance, can kill or permanently damage a child.) As long as your GP has your up-to-date address, you'll automatically be sent appointments for your baby's immunisations. You can help your baby cope with having an injection by holding him close to your body (studies show babies are less stressed if held close by their parents), letting him a suck a dummy, breast or finger, and by talking or singing calmly to him while it's happening.

Many babies, in the twenty-four hours or so after their immunisations, get a redness or swelling where they had the injection (it's tender, so be gentle). They may also have a fever, so give them Calpol or baby ibuprofen in the dose advised by your GP or nurse. Often this means a disturbed night after the jabs.

Reasons to give up smoking now

To quit, contact Action on Smoking and Health (for details see **Contacts**.

If you want to do one thing for your baby's welfare, give up smoking. Every year 17,000 children are admitted to hospital because their parents smoke, and smoking is directly linked to cot death.

IF YOU SMOKE, YOUR CHILD IS MORE LIKELY TO HAVE:

- Coughs and colds
- Chest infections
- Asthma
- Ear infections
- Parents who die young

If you can't give up, don't smoke around your baby and ideally make your house a smoke-free zone.

Basic First Aid

As a parent, you're going to have to deal with quite a few bumps and cuts at the very least. You might want to go for an evening or day of First Aid training for your own peace of mind and to learn some basic skills. To find one contact your local branch of the British Red Cross (www.redcross.org.uk). Make sure your babysitters know where you keep the First Aid kit. It's a good idea to keep one in the car too.

What to do if your baby ...

... IS BLEEDING

You have to press on the wound and keep the injured bit raised (so the blood drains back into the body and not out of the cut). Cover the wound with a sterile dressing and a bandage, then get medical help. If it's a smaller cut or scratch, just wash it with soap and warm water and dab it dry with a clean towel, then put a plaster on. If there is a fragment of something in the wound, take it out if you can do so easily. Otherwise get a doctor to do it.

... BASHES HIS HEAD

Mostly babies who bump their heads are fine. But if you can't rouse your baby, call an ambulance. If he loses consciousness but wakes up quickly, take him to the doctor even if he seems fine when he wakes up. If he wasn't unconscious, seems normal and is not bleeding, watch him carefully for a couple of days after the bump: drowsiness, vomiting, looking very pale or deep sleeping (when you can't wake him up) mean you should contact a doctor immediately. Putting a cold compress – a bag of peas wrapped in a tea towel will do – on the bump can bring down the swelling. It's normal for a bump to look quite dramatic.

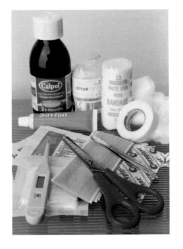

YOU SHOULD HAVE A **FIRST AID KIT** IN THE HOUSE CONTAINING:

- ⊙ **Plasters**
- ⊙ **Sterile dressings**
- ⊙ **Bandages**
- ⊙ **Antiseptic ointment**
- ⊙ **Cotton wool**
- ⊙ **Small scissors and tweezers**
- ⊙ **Adhesive tape (to hold bandages in place)**
- ⊙ **Infant fever medicine such as infant paracetamol or infant ibuprofen**
- ⊙ **A thermometer (digital is best)**

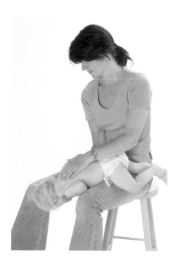

Make sure the baby is facing head downwards.

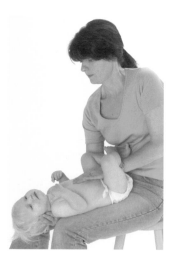

If the obstruction does not clear, call an ambulance immediately.

... CHOKES

Your baby will turn blue and make strangulated noises if he's choking. Don't turn him upside down or shake him.

BEFORE YOU CALL AN AMBULANCE:

1 | Lay him face down along your forearm or across your knee and give him five sharp slaps in the middle of his back. Check between each slap to see if the obstruction has cleared.
2 | If he's still choking, turn him face up on your arm or across your knee. Use one finger to check for any obvious obstructions inside his mouth.
3 | If there are none, put two fingers on the lower half of his breastbone and press down sharply five times.
4 | Check his mouth again and see if you can take out whatever it is he's choking on.
5 | Call an ambulance if it's still there, and keep on giving the slaps/thrusts while you're waiting.
6 | If he's unconscious, *see page 170* for what to do.

... SEEMS TO HAVE BROKEN A BONE

A bone in the arm or leg may be broken if it's obviously causing him pain, is swelling up and looks 'wrong' – at an odd angle, bruised, possibly with a wound where the broken bit is. If you think his neck or spine might be hurt, *don't move him* and call an ambulance right away. If you move him, you might do even more serious damage (you can cause paralysis). If it's not his spine or neck that seems damaged, but you can't easily move him without obviously hurting him even more, call an ambulance anyway. If you have to move him, be super gentle and try not to let the broken bit flop around (pad it with a blanket or clothes if necessary). Give him lots of comfort and take him to A&E straight away.

... HAS SOMETHING STUCK UP HIS NOSE OR IN HIS EAR

This is very common as babies start to explore the world and themselves. If you think he has put something up his nose or in his ear and it's not obviously incredibly easy to pull it out (for example a pencil with a lot protruding) don't touch it - you could push it further in. Take him to A&E where a doctor will remove the object with forceps.

... GETS A BURN

You have to cool the burn quickly and get any clothes off it before the burned bit starts to swell. Take clothes off the area and run it under cold water for ten minutes (even if your baby is screaming – cold water is good pain relief, and may stop the burn area getting bigger). Give him pain medicine (Calpol or baby ibuprofen) straight away (even small burns are extraordinarily painful). Don't put any creams or anything else on it, but do cover the burn with cling film if you have some – other dressings may stick to the skin and will be painful to remove. 'All burns in babies need to be seen by a doctor,' says emergency medicine specialist Dr Liza Keating, 'but anything you are worried about, or a burn that is failing to settle, needs to be seen at A&E.'

... GETS AN ELECTRIC SHOCK

An electric shock can stop your baby breathing, and may stop his heart. Switch off the current at the mains before you touch your baby (or you could get electrocuted too, in which case you'd be unable to save him). Stand on something like a telephone directory and push the source of the shock away with a broom. Start any resuscitation necessary and call an ambulance.

... GETS SOMETHING IN HIS EYE

If something gets in your baby's eye, wash it out with water and try to stop him rubbing his eye. If it was something liquid (spray cleaner, for instance) flush out the eye with lukewarm water – pour water into the eye, with your baby lying on his back – for several minutes. This will be stressful, as most babies will be yelling and thrashing, but you must do it. If you can't make it completely better, go to your GP.

... SWALLOWS SOMETHING HE SHOULDN'T

If your baby swallows a small, smooth object (a cherry stone, say) and doesn't seem bothered, it's likely to just come out the other end. If it's sharp, or causes him to choke, you need to get medical help immediately *(see choking, above)*.

If he's swallowed something you know or suspect is poisonous and seems ill, call an ambulance. Don't try to make him vomit. Even if he seems fine, call your doctor, hospital or NHS DIRECT (0845 46 47) straight away (sometimes you get delayed reactions). Bring the substance with you to the hospital/doctor if you can.

If your baby is unconscious

FIRST THINGS TO
KNOW ARE:

If you really can't wake your baby up, he is probably unconscious.
Look, listen and feel for breathing, paying particular attention to
his tummy – is there any movement? If you can't detect breathing you
need to open his airways and help him breathe by breathing into his
lungs for him. If his heart has slowed down or stopped, you also need
to resuscitate him using 'chest compressions'.

⊙ **You have to do something
to resuscitate him before
you call an ambulance.
Get someone to call the
ambulance while you do
this, if you have someone
with you. A minute of
your immediate efforts
could save his life.**

If your baby is breathing but unconscious, call an ambulance
immediately. He could choke on his tongue or vomit, so stand and
cradle him with his tummy against yours and his head lower than
his chest so that his airway is open. Keep checking his pulse and
breathing until help arrives.

ARTIFICIAL VENTILATION ('MOUTH TO MOUTH'):

If he's not breathing, you need to breathe into his lungs for him so he
gets oxygen:

⊙ **Have your baby next to
you if possible when you
call the ambulance
because the person on the
end of the phone will be
trained to help you until
the ambulance gets there.**

1 | Lie him on his back. Put one finger under his chin and your other
hand on his head. Tilt his head back to open the airway.

2 | Remove anything you can clearly see in his throat that might be
choking him.

3 | Put your lips over his mouth and nose and breathe into his lungs
until you see his chest rise. Take your lips off and let his chest fall
back down.

4 | Do this for a minute. Ideally you want to be giving him *one*
breath every *three* seconds (breathe into his nose and mouth,
count 1, 2, 3 and breathe again, 1, 2, 3 breathe ...)

5 | Look for any signs of a circulation. This tells you how well his
heart is beating. It can be very difficult to feel for a pulse unless
you've had training. Instead look for any movement, coughing or
breathing. If your baby is unresponsive, floppy and pale, there is
either no circulation or an inadequate circulation. If there are no
signs of a circulation or you are at all unsure, start chest
compressions ('unnecessary' chest compressions are almost
never damaging).

CHEST COMPRESSIONS

If he has no signs of an adequate circulation, you have to help his
heart to beat.

1 | Put two fingers on his lower breastbone – this is a finger's
breadth below an imaginary line joining his nipples.

2 | Press down firmly with the tips of these two fingers (the chest
should go down about an inch where you press) five times, rapidly.

3 | Tilt his head, lift his chin and give one mouth-to-mouth breath *(as above)*.

4 | Press down firmly again, five times rapidly.

5 | Keep alternating the breathing and chest compressions until help arrives (five compressions to one breath).

For more detailed information about life support, try the Resuscitation Council website's paediatric basic life-support section at www.resus.org.uk.

Basic child safety

All babies and children get hurt from time to time, but there are some practical things you can do to minimise the chances that it will be serious. Asphyxia (choking, strangulation, suffocation) is the third most common cause of accidental death in children in the UK (after road-traffic accidents and house fires). Other common causes of injury to children are burns, poisoning and falls.

THERE ARE A FEW THINGS YOU CAN DO TO MAKE YOUR HOME SAFER:

- Store all drugs, painkillers, medicines, cosmetics, alcohol and vitamin pills in a cabinet with a child-resistant lock.
- Keep all household and gardening chemicals – including cleaning products – in a cupboard with child-resistant locks.
- Screw child-resistant lids on tight and never put anything your child shouldn't drink in a drinks bottle.
- Put plug guards on open sockets and check your appliance flexes are not worn or dangling where a baby can grab them.
- Install stair gates and window locks on upstairs windows (or any with a drop) to stop the window opening far enough for your baby or child to get out. Check that your baby can't fit through the railings on your balcony or landing.
- Keep choking/suffocation hazards out of reach. Only let your baby have age-appropriate toys – small toys or parts are common chokers (if a toy is small enough to fit inside the tube of a loo roll it is a hazard). Don't leave your baby alone when eating, and don't give him hard-textured nuts or boiled sweets to chomp until he's much bigger (four or five). Broken balloon pieces, coins, batteries and buttons are all common chokers, and string, ribbon, elastic and plastic bags can choke, strangle or suffocate a baby or child.

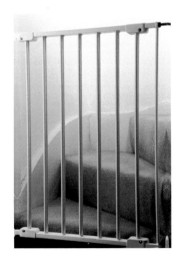

Child-resistant locks prevent little fingers from getting at the contents of your cupboards.

A stair gate is essential once your baby starts crawling.

- By far the most common cause of scalds to babies and toddlers is hot drinks. A mug of tea can scald a baby fifteen minutes after it's made, so keep all hot drinks way out of reach. Turn the temperature of your water down to 49°C (120°F). At 65–75°C (150–160°F) a small child will get a third-degree burn in less than two seconds. Ideally keep your baby in the high chair when you're cooking, always point saucepan handles towards the back of the stove and use back rings where possible (even a baby who can't walk may pull himself up and grab a handle). Watch out for kettles, irons (and their flexes), candles and barbecues.

For more information on child safety, see **Contacts**.

- Fit smoke detectors. Eighty per cent of fire-related deaths happen in house fires, so also get a fire extinguisher and fire blanket and think about your exit routes.

Pet safety

You are not the only ones whose world is about to be rocked by a new family member. The last thing you want is a jealous dog, or a cat who decides the Moses basket (ideally with a nice warm infant in it) is her new bed. In general there's no reason to avoid having pets and babies in the same house (unless you own a crocodile or a savage, grudge-bearing pooch). But always be vigilant and take precautions: make sure your pet is healthy and has been wormed, de-flead and vaccinated before your baby arrives. Don't assume your pet is 'safe' just because he's never done anything dodgy: never let your pet and baby sleep in the same room, and supervise your baby's interaction with your pet at all times.

DOG TIPS

Get your dog fully trained before your baby arrives. A dog's training and individual temperament are more important than its breed. Some doggie-behaviour experts advise playing your dog tapes of a baby crying (three to four times a day for a week, gradually increasing the volume to get him used to the disruption ahead), though this could be bad for your own sanity. You could also get someone to bring a blanket or piece of clothing home from the hospital that your baby has been wearing and let the dog sniff it so that he gets used to the baby's smell before he has to live with it. If you are inundated with visitors, keep the dog somewhere quiet so he does not get overexcited or wound up.

CAT TIPS

The main danger with cats (apart from the odd scratch or nip when a tail is yanked) is that they like sleeping on anything warm. If left alone with your baby your cat could suffocate him by sleeping on top of him. Always be sure that, if you leave your baby sleeping, there is a closed door between him and the cat (and the cat can't get in the window). You can also buy 'cat nets' that go over cots and stop a cat from settling on the baby. Cat toys are choking hazards like anything else, and finally, curious babies often get their heads stuck in cat flaps, so be vigilant.

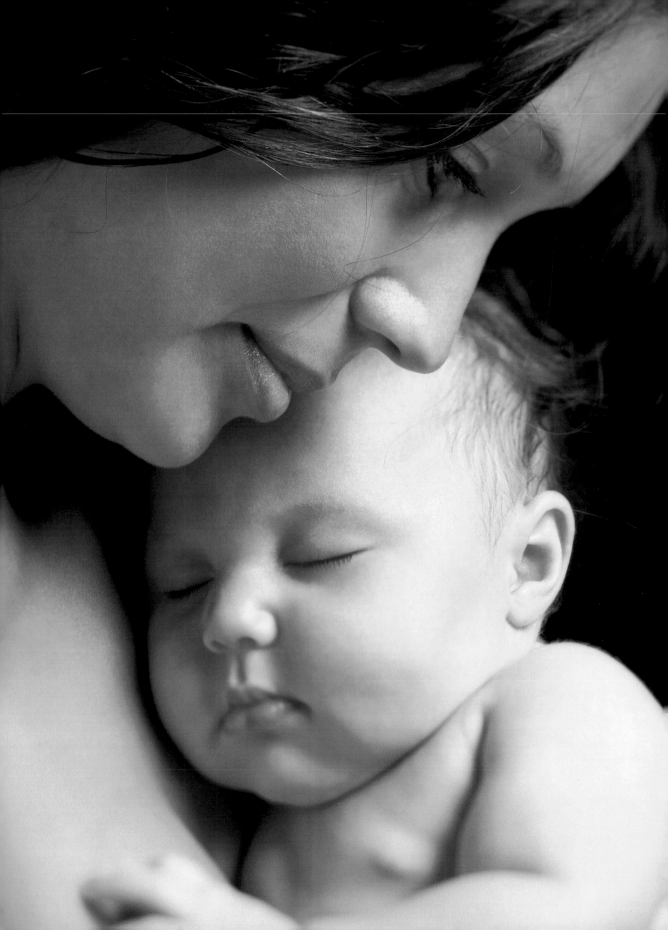

live

Your relationship and identity post-baby

I find it impossible to suppress a hollow laugh when I hear of a couple deciding to have a baby to 'cement the relationship'. It's true: having a baby, or babies, can certainly make you acutely aware of how much you love and adore one another. It's an incredibly special thing to do together. And your baby really is the ultimate, miraculous manifestation of your love and commitment (and the ultimate shared goal). But on a practical, day-to-day level, babies can test even the most solid partnership to the limit. So it's worth working out how to keep things on track (one word: babysitters).

Sex (mostly, lack of …)

You go from Wonderbras to bras with milk stains and flaps; from long, loving lie-ins to 5 a.m. wake-ups and nights that are sleepless for wholly different reasons. 'The effect of a baby on a relationship is huge,' says parenting expert Lorraine Thomas. 'Many women say to me that sex is top of their partner's agenda and bottom of their to-do list.'

Sex is clearly not just about physical stuff like sleep deprivation, stitches and breastfeeding. Adjusting to your new roles can actually be quite a turn-off. And not just for women – 'I think he sees me as a mother now instead of his lover,' says Hannah, mother of Nico, six months. What's more, if you haven't been to the loo unaccompanied for six months and spend your days elbow deep in poo and mushed-up carrot, you may not feel like slipping into a negligee of an evening.

'You go from Wonderbras to bras with milk stains and flaps; from long, loving lie-ins to 5 a.m. wake-ups and nights that are sleepless for wholly different reasons.'

Your baby *will* sleep more one day, your stitches *will* heal, you may go back to some kind of work, and you will at some point regain at least a vague sense of who you are. But at first, it has to be said, motherhood can be a fabulous method of contraception (don't bank on this though).

Your relationship

'It can be so, so easy to put your own relationship on the back-burner during the intensely demanding early days – and leave it there,' writes Relate counsellor Elizabeth Martyn in her book *Baby Shock!* In essence, she (and virtually every psychologist, psychiatrist and family therapist in existence) has one thing to say on this subject: *don't*.

In 2002 there were 149,335 children of divorced parents in the UK. It's no accident that a quarter of these children were under four. According to the relationship research and training organisation One Plus One, studies generally show that the most difficult hurdle for couples is the birth of their first baby. I'm not trying to scare you here, but to show you it's worth putting some effort into your relationship, even in the thick of new-baby madness, because ideally you want your baby to grow up with two parents who do not require either gritted teeth or a mediator to communicate.

But first let's be realistic. You are neither unusual nor failing as a couple, if you:

- Don't have sex for months (or only have disappointing sex)
- Put each other's needs way down the list
- Bicker more than ever before
- Shout more than ever before, or start shouting if you never did before
- Feel zero enthusiasm for romance
- Feel like you're in different worlds
- Wish you had your 'old relationship' back

All these things are normal for new parents. But most of us wake up one day and realise we still adore and fancy each other (often more than ever). At this point we decide to *have another baby*.

One survey found that eight out of ten new mothers preferred sleep to sex. The other two out of ten presumably hired night nannies, wore earplugs or were lying. When you're three stone overweight, have boobs like medicine balls, a vagina full of stitches and have not cleaned your teeth for two weeks – let alone touched a bottle of shampoo – sex is unlikely to top your agenda.

Sleep deprivation is the main relationship-problem culprit. Most couples find ways to cope with it: we bring the baby to bed with us (something one Relate counsellor calls 'a very effective chastity belt'), we sleep in separate rooms, we take turns to take the baby out and give the other a 'break'. 'For the first three months we slept in shifts,' says Devon, mother of Ariel, five months. 'I went to bed from 8 p.m. to 2 a.m. and then my husband went to bed and I stayed up with the baby. We put a bed in the living room.' These strategies, while helpful in terms of survival, can distance even the most loved-up couple. 'We don't have much of a physical relationship at the moment,' says Melissa, mother of Raphael, nine months. 'Part of the problem is that we don't sleep together at night as one or other of us is usually with the baby and the other sleeps in another bed.'

Your sleep-crisis arrangements should be temporary (if they're still going on after about six months, you may want to address your baby's sleep habits head-on). The effect on your sex life, however, may be more long-lasting. 'The lack of sleep means we have no sex,' says Gina, mother of Felix, eight months. 'Given any time alone we end up cuddling and going to sleep.'

Still, at least they're cuddling. Some new parents rarely even touch, let alone have sex. Finding (small, relatively easy) ways to connect, sex or no sex, bed sharing or no bed sharing, is a really good idea.

HERE ARE FOUR WAYS TO BRIDGE THE DIVIDE:

- Make the effort to touch. Kiss, hold hands, have a quick back rub or a hug whenever you can: any physical contact is good. A baby can quite literally come between you.
- Listen to one another, and try to put yourself in the other person's shoes. OK, so your day involved a teething baby, twenty-five squitty nappies and an eyeful of pee; what was his stressful day like for him? Stress and exhaustion one-upmanship, while tempting, is never helpful.
- Make eye contact. It sounds silly, but so many couples don't just stop touching, they stop looking at each other. When you fell in love you probably spent hours gazing into each other's eyes. You can't do this now without falling asleep; but you can, when you kiss goodbye in the morning and hello at night, look into one another's eyes. It does make a difference.
- Get a babysitter. In the first few months this is unlikely to happen. But once you're able to stay awake beyond 8 p.m., it's vital to *go out* regularly, just the two of you. It doesn't have to be any big deal – even a walk together can be bonding. And, as the Relate book puts it, 'It isn't selfish or indulgent to take time for yourselves … it's essential.'

Men and sex

Your beautiful, vibrant lover has turned into an unhinged, big-knicker-wearing psycho. It can be very hard suddenly to feel as if your sex life is over, possibly for good. And that you're bad for even *thinking* about sex. And that if you touch her, she'll think you're thinking about sex, and bat you away. And that all she cares about now is the baby. And that, anyway, you'll probably *hurt* her if you try to have sex. And that it was sex that got you into this mess in the first place. And that, when you think about it, you don't actually feel much like having sex either. Yes, resuming sex after childbirth can take a long time for men too.

EIGHT RULES FOR SEXUAL SURVIVAL:

1 | Make masturbation your friend.
2 | Reassure your partner that she's beautiful. She may be five stone heavier, with handfuls of spare skin, stretch marks, bulging veins and red-rimmed eyes but she is, to you, beautiful – OK? Certainly, telling her this a lot is a very good idea if you ever want those big knickers to come off.
3 | Be patient. If you had squeezed a rugby ball out of your arse (after nine months of unfeasible swelling and hours of agonising pains) – in living memory, let alone a few weeks or months ago – would you want someone putting something up there? I think not.
4 | Avoid blame. Everyone lies about sex. The vast majority of couples actually have little or no sex in the months (and sometimes longer) after having a baby. You are not alone, your partner is not unreasonable, and if you are patient and loving, sex will, one day, come back.
5 | Stay connected. See the four ways to bridge the divide *(above)*.
6 | Do not ring the six-week check in red on your calendar: it may be technically possible to have intercourse at this point, but for many women it's utterly off the agenda.
7 | Have a no-sex clause. If you're finding you don't even touch any more because you get rebuffed, make an agreement that you will touch - massage, stroke, whatever - but that no penetrative sex will happen. *Stick to this* or the whole thing becomes pointless and she'll never let you touch her again. This is a vital step to reclaiming some intimacy if sex is not happening.
8 | Be prepared to talk about sex. If you can communicate how you feel - in a non-judgmental way, not in the bedroom, and not after you've just been rejected - it can really help you both get through this.

Sex: some practicalities

When you do both feel like getting back in the saddle, there are some small considerations you might like to bear in mind:

- Do you want another baby? If not, don't rely on breastfeeding, a lack of periods or any teenage-type withdrawal methods as contraception. Many couples end up with extremely closely timed first and second children because they do not realise they're fertile (duh!). You may not have *had* a period, but who's to say you've not just released your first post-baby ovum?

- Make sure sex is OK'd at your six-week check. Your GP will be able to tell you whether it is at least safe to have a go.
- Take the whole thing very gingerly. If you have given birth vaginally, you may still be surprisingly tender around there. If you have torn badly during the birth, you can be (slightly) sore for ages. I, over a year after giving birth to Ted, am still sore. My tear was really bad, but still ... it's possible. Gentle stretching is good for any scars in your vagina – though this is hardly an aphrodisiac – but do go slow.
- Indulge in plenty of foreplay for obvious reasons (lubrication and enthusiasm being the main ones) ...
- ... but go easy on the boobs if you're breastfeeding: they can be extraordinarily oversensitive, which is a potentially catastrophic turn-off. Incidentally – brace yourself here – they may spurt milk on orgasm.
- Try lubricants. You can buy them from any chemist and they can really help the first few goes at sex.
- Try other stuff. If penetrative sex is just too hard (literally), try oral sex, masturbation, massage and other nice things until you're up to the whole hog again.
- Have a few drinks – the whole thing is likely to be easier. And if it isn't, you're more likely to laugh about it.
- Dim the lights. Most men don't give a hoot – they're just delighted that it's an option at all – but even the most secure, gung-ho new mother can be inhibited by the sight of her own blue-veined baps leaking milk on to the pillow, or the fact that she must forklift her bellies into position. Think candlelight.
- Get some nice knickers. Squeezing into posh knickers that are three sizes too small will make you feel worse about your body, and most post-baby knickers are large, stained and horrific. Buy some sexy pants in your new, scarily capacious (sorry, 'curvaceous') size.
- Remember size doesn't matter. Yours, not his. You may feel you're the size of the Mersey tunnel down there, but you really aren't. It's amazing how vaginas spring back after childbirth. And even if you are somewhat more stretched than before, post-baby sex is generally a cause for vast celebration for most men, regardless of the details. If you are doing your pelvic floor exercises regularly, your elasticity will come back. Well, up to a point. No one said having babies was easy.

The floodgates

Sex after childbirth can be a hugely emotional event, not just because you're both vastly relieved to be doing it again. Be prepared for a few false starts. You may be raring to go, then just be unable to face it when, ahem, push comes to shove. Both of you need to be prepared to stop if it's all too much. Expect some big emotions: some women find having sex brings some of the memories of childbirth back. And communicate – many men are terrified of hurting their partners, having seen what went on down there. Be sensitive to each other and, again, take things very slowly.

A few other common sources of new-parent tension

Madonna and child syndrome

You wake up one day and you're a mother. In a flash, all your desire, love, sensual pleasure, hopes, dreams and wonderment have transferred from your lovely man to your infinitely lovelier infant. It's like falling under some powerful, woo-woo spell: you now know that, given some disaster scenario, you'd trample your partner's struggling body to get to your baby. None of this actually means you love your man less (you probably love him more, if anything). But something has definitely shifted.

Your partner, meanwhile, is probably hovering somewhere in the background saying, 'Er, could I help, do you think?' He may feel equally passionate about his newborn, but his hormones are not telling him to grasp the baby to his breast and keep her there to the exclusion of everyone else until she's at least twenty-one.

'I think he feels pushed out,' says Gina, mother of Felix, eight months. 'I don't think he enjoys being a parent as much as I do. I want him to be as happy as I am, and I don't think he is.' 'Imagine,' suggests the Relate book, 'if anyone other than your baby moved in with you and one of you fell in love.' There'd be ructions, that's for sure.

Getting territorial (insisting on doing it all yourself, hovering over your partner barking instructions or criticisms as he tries to change a nappy) can really exacerbate the distance between you. Instead, try to:

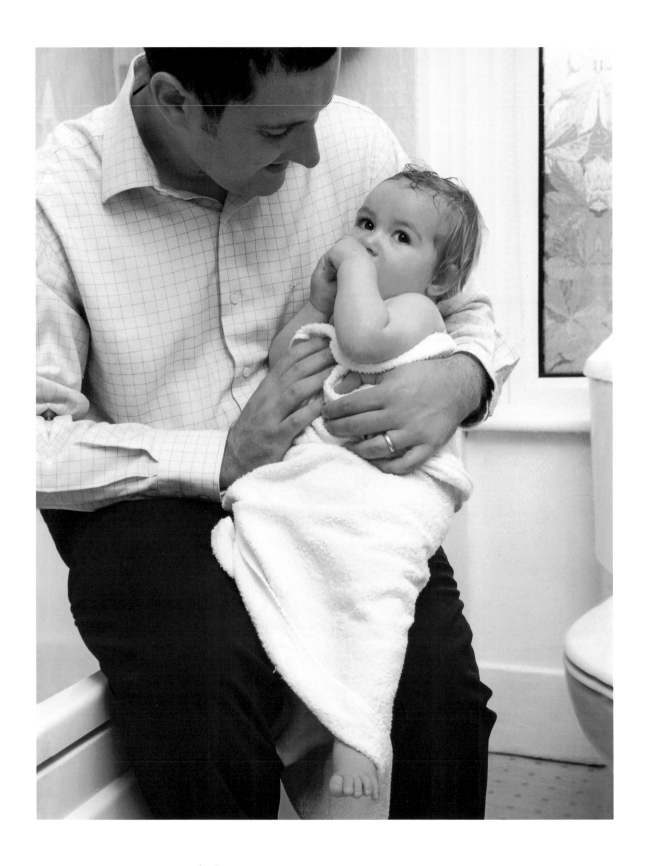

- Share some feeds (you can occasionally express milk, if you're breastfeeding, so your partner can feed the baby with a bottle).
- Leave the room while your partner is in charge of the baby so you are not tempted to interfere (and so you get a break, and therefore a small, perhaps momentary, sense of perspective).
- Divide up baby-care tasks so you each get time to be 'in charge' of your baby. Bath time, for instance, could be Daddy's – without Mummy barking orders and peeking through the keyhole to check the baby isn't drowning.
- Quell the urge to criticise. Different is not necessarily worse and your way is not always best. (If you can't quell this urge, leave the room.)
- Praise each other a lot ('What a fabulous nappy-change, darling. You're a pro!' 'Did I mention, my love, that you are a breast-feeding goddess?')

Birth shock

A terrible birthing ordeal can leave you both shell-shocked. Months after childbirth many women have flashbacks and show signs of genuine trauma while many men, at some point during a difficult birth, believe that their partner, or baby, or both, are going to die. Hardly a relaxing memory. Difficult experiences of childbirth have been linked to post-traumatic stress disorder and postnatal depression, and can really drive couples apart.

YOU COULD TRY THE FOLLOWING:

- Write down what happened (both of you). Who did what? Who said what? How long did various stages take? How did it feel, both emotionally and physically? What shocked you? What didn't? What was amazing?
- Sit down with your midwife a few weeks or months after the event, with your notes, to get explanations for the grey areas and confusing bits.
- Talk to your midwife or health visitor about counselling. Don't compare your story to others – if it was upsetting for you, that's a good enough reason to get help, whatever happened.
- Get support from Birth Crisis, an organisation set up by birth expert Sheila Kitzinger to help women who have had a difficult experience of childbirth. Find out more at www.sheilakitzinger.com.

Role changes

If one of you (usually the woman) is suddenly at home, not earning or earning little, and the other has become the breadwinner, it's easy to feel you've suddenly been catapulted back into the 1950s. Many new fathers at this point get so-called 'provider fever' – an anxiety about money and this new sense of vast responsibility. Many mummies, meanwhile, are not completely comfortable in this new world of cooking, cleaning, laundry and other mind-numbing household chores. Such life changes can lead to tension. If you can sort out a budget and do some conscious financial planning, this may help you get to grips with the financial drain of your changed earning status. But the domestic stuff is a different matter.

'It's easy to feel you've suddenly been catapulted back into the 1950s.'

A FEW TIPS FOR WORKING FATHERS:

- Let your partner know when you're going to be home and stick to it religiously. We pace ourselves: if you're not back when you said you'd be, we may lose it. This is just the way it is. Ten minutes to a frazzled mother at the end of the day is ten hours to normal people. If you are late, expect to find her standing at the door ready to hurl a wailing baby at you, rugby style, as you cross the threshold.
- Make sure you do stuff with the baby without your partner: you need to keep involved and hands-on, even if you're not there during the day, or she'll entirely take over, then resent you for it (and you'll miss out badly).
- Make bolstering gestures: phone her during the day just to ask how it's going (expect to be shouted/sobbed at sometimes). If at all possible, be prepared to let your work suffer a bit at first: if you can very occasionally just down tools and go home when she's really at the end of her tether, she will feel you at least have some appreciation of what she's going through.
- Do your share of domestic chores (see below).

- Draw up (yes, on paper – be anal) some arrangement on who does what, how often and when.

- Stick to this.

- Be realistic. Hiring a cleaner once a week, while a vast bonus if you can afford it, will not remove the bulk of daily domestic tasks – laundry, picking things up, putting things away, cooking, shopping, bill-paying …

- At least for the first six weeks after the baby is born accept that the father, as the one with no boobs, rocketing hormones or stitches, will take the brunt of domesticity. Be very, very clear about this, preferably in advance.

- If this is not possible, do all you can to get help with these things.

Domestic chores

How could anyone so small have such a seismic impact on your house? One recent survey found that 'getting a cleaner and having fewer domestic chores' beat 'spending more quality time with my partner' for new mothers, hands down. Looking after babies and small children is extremely hard work. It is utterly unreasonable to think that the one at home should be responsible for *all* the housework too. You'll have your own tolerance levels on this one, but if you're not happy with the division of labour (or have the feeling that thirty years of feminist thought have apparently vanished in a puff of baby powder), it's vital to communicate about this, and come to some agreements.

Agreeing on the fundamentals

Relate counsellors say fundamental differences in outlook are responsible for much relationship tension in new parents. You think you're rowing about the untidy kitchen, but really you're rowing about whether mothers should work outside the home/fathers should be disciplinarian/children should be seen and not heard …

To start with, sit down and discuss what being a 'good mother' and a 'good father' really mean to you. Being at home? Providing financially? Discipline? Tolerance? The more you can talk – and reach agreements and compromises – the less likely you are to row at the drop of a hat. If such talks end in World War Three, getting help from a third party (a counsellor) before it all gets out of hand can be genuinely useful.

Since we're talking fundamentals, here's another: get your wills drawn up. When you become parents, it becomes important to sort out what would happen to your baby if something happened to you. It's horrific to consider, but you're officially grown-ups now and have to do this sort of thing.

Some tips for talking

- Make some time to talk – even fifteen minutes will do – when you are neither speechless with exhaustion, nor hungry, nor reeling from your latest shouting match.
- Take turns to listen to each other, uninterrupted, for a set amount of time (five or ten minutes each is good). It's amazing what you learn if you're forced to listen.
- Reflect. Don't leap to respond, even if what the other person says makes you livid. You're aiming to end up with a better grasp of the other person's feelings, not to 'win' some ongoing debate.

- Try to agree a solution that satisfies you both (but be realistic: if you compromise too much, the issues won't be resolved, they'll be shelved for later.)
- Turn off the TV. Even if it's only once a week, try to have an evening where you sit down together and talk, or read to one another, or cook and eat a meal together.
- Go to bed very early once in a while – if you don't crash out, it can be very bonding to have time awake in bed together (sex or no sex).

You

OK, so I should be going on about 'me' time here. It is, indeed, crucial for you to get some time away from your baby to shop, sit in a bookshop, read the paper in a café, go for a swim or just walk unaccompanied by someone who may, at any moment, need feeding or changing. But the reality is that in the first few months, when you need it most, you're usually too shattered to care about 'me' time. You don't know who 'me' is any more, and any time you get you're likely to spend asleep, or simply lying, dazed, on the bedroom floor wondering how you'll ever muster the energy to pull on your jeans.

Don't beat yourself up about any of this. Use any spare time you have to do whatever will help you survive at that point (sleep is fine). Talking to girlfriends is always reaffirming and may remind you that you are – or once were at least – a sentient human being, not just a crazed milk-machine. I can also recommend solo trips to the cinema with only an undemanding bag of Maltesers for company: excellent down time for shattered new mothers.

Who am I?

You may slip into parenthood without a hitch, wondering what everyone else is making such a fuss about. Or you may find the world has undergone a seismic shift. 'I've been surprised how important family feels, the threads and connection of blood and care,' says Melissa, mother of Raphael. 'The perspective I now have on everyday people has changed: people who fight wars, who die, who kill, commit crimes, sacrifice themselves – they are all mothers' sons and daughters. Somewhere, perhaps their mothers feel the way I do about my son.'

This new perspective can also give you a renewed sense of your own value. 'I feel how sad it would be if I died now,' says Aishah, mother of Reyhana, six months. 'How terrible it would be to leave my baby without a mother.' You may also see things in yourself that you've never seen before. As Laura, mother of Reuben, four months, puts it, 'I have never been so impressed with myself.'

Finally, you never know how a baby will affect you or your relationship. But you can guarantee one thing: there'll be a few surprises. 'I gained a relationship after introducing Tola to my first boyfriend,' says Madeleine. 'We first met when I was seventeen. He came to visit Tola and we all fell in love. We plan to be married soon.'

Deeper love

For more information on how your baby will affect your relationships, see **Contacts**.

So it's not all bad news, honest. Parenthood doesn't just unite your genes and your priorities, it can also bring out new, and at times amazing, qualities in you and your relationship. 'There is the tiredness, and the disagreements about little things,' says Melissa, mother of Raphael, 'but generally I feel we have graduated to another level of commitment and deep love.' A side-effect of this is that many of us become genuinely afraid that our partners will leave us, or die. This is part of your mutual graduation to parenthood and it can be hugely positive (death-anxieties aside). And all this deep love can really be quite sexy once the exhaustion abates.

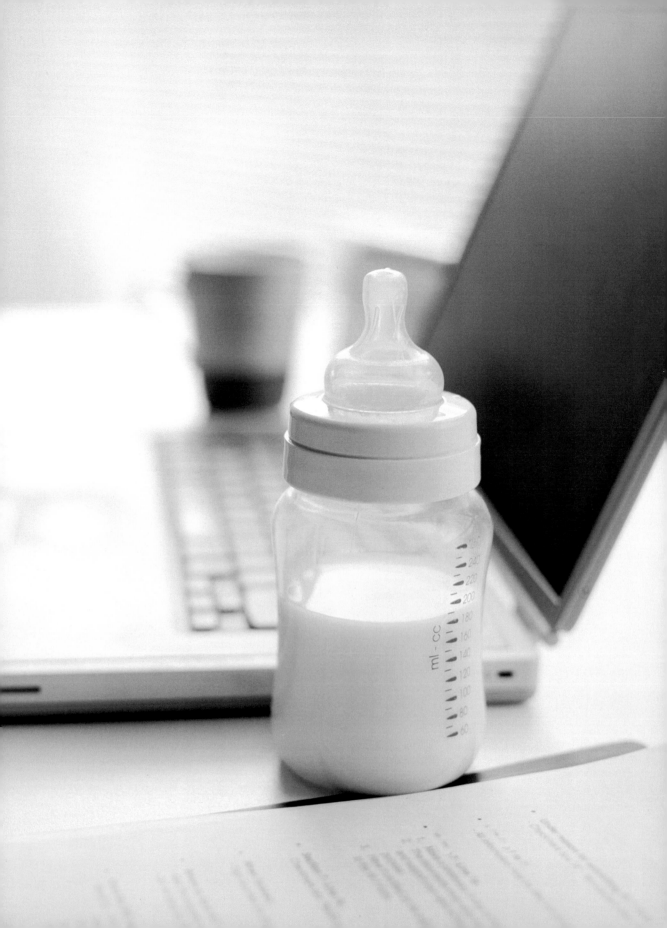

work

That elusive 'work-life balance' and how to get, well ... at least *something* like it

It's a fact: you *can* now have it all. The only problem is you'll probably go loony in the process. Working out how to balance your career and your parenting life is no picnic. In fact the whole notion that it's completely do-able if you just make 'proper' plans is a bit suspect, if you ask me. No matter how well you've planned things, there's bound to be some doubt, ambivalence, tension or longing (one way or the other) from time to time. However, if you're even to have a stab at arranging your work and home life to suit your family best, there are a few issues you really should consider.

Nowadays the working parent's options have never been more abundant. You can become an 'at-home' mum or dad, go back to work part-time, flexitime, job-share or full-time; you can divide parental care equally, hire night nannies, day nannies, maternity nurses, au pairs or child-minders, or choose from a whole range of nurseries. You're legally entitled to paid time off work for having a baby, and time off if your baby is sick or your childcare arrangements implode. It all sounds like the simplest thing in the world.

So why, then, do eight out of ten mothers who have recently returned to work feel they've got the 'work–life balance' wrong? Why do seventy per cent of them feel guilty for leaving their baby, and more than half feel they're being pulled in too many directions? Here are a few issues you might want to explore if you are to give that elusive 'work–life' balance your best shot.

Giving up work

Working mothers often hanker after full-time motherhood. Full-time mothers often long to flee to an office. But one thing virtually all experienced mothers say about formulating post-baby work plans is wait and see. 'You tend to be much more hard-headed about your plans for returning to work before you have your baby,' says BBC presenter Sophie Raworth, mother of Ella, now one. 'Once Ella was born, I found the idea of going back to work so much harder than I ever thought I would. I felt so torn.'

'Full-time mothers often long to flee to an office.'

Looking after babies and small children can be delightful and fulfilling work. But it's definitely work. Exactly how delightful and fulfilling it is for you will depend on your personality, outlook, circumstances and, to some extent, baby. It is rarely, however, the 'easy' option.

Money
You may scoff at the notion of choice: you have to go back to work because if you don't the mortgage company will repossess your home. If this makes you feel pressurised, the first thing to do is a budget (childcare can eat up a huge chunk of your earnings, so whether it's financially worth it may well be a realistic question to ask).

- A full-time nursery place for a child under two is about £141 a week in England – that's over £7,300 a year (it rises to about £10,000 a year in inner London).
- A full-time place with a childminder for a child under two in England is about £127 a week, or over £6,600 a year (around £200 a week in inner London).
- A full-time qualified nanny can cost more than many of us earn (you have to pay their tax and national insurance too).

Working anxiety

In general, working-parent anxiety comes in two basic forms: 'will my baby be safe?' and 'will childcare harm my baby's development?' Let's start with the latter.

WILL CHILDCARE HARM MY BABY?

Studies pop up from time to time saying your child will either be more or less intelligent/damaged/sociopathic than others if you leave him with someone else for all or part of the week. None of these are conclusive and they certainly don't make particularly helpful bedtime reading for working parents. The vast majority of children in this country spend part of their time being cared for by someone other than their parents. The one thing that does seem clear is that it's the *quality* of the care your baby gets when you're not there that matters most of all. One-to-one care from a trusted adult until at least the age of two is supposed to be the ideal, but a good nursery is plainly better than a crappy nanny or a bonkers at-home mother who wishes she was at work. Ultimately you have to work out something that *feels right* for you and can work for your family, practically, financially and emotionally.

WILL MY BABY BE SAFE WITH SOMEONE ELSE?

I don't want to come over all Obi-Wan Kenobi 'feel the force' here, but the truth is that your instinct holds the true answer to this one.

When I took my first baby, Isabella, to nursery for the first time, I sobbed all the way home, sat at my kitchen table weeping for five minutes then ran back to get her. She was fine. But I cancelled the nursery place right there: I just couldn't do it. At the time I was embarrassed at how pathetic I was, but looking back on it, with three babies' worth of childcare arrangements under my belt, I now realise that I was *completely right*: that first nursery, while not actually dangerous, was not a very loving environment (as other nurseries I've since used have been). I was following my instincts, even if I didn't know it at the time.

If you don't have a really positive instinct about your baby's care, ask yourself why. And be honest with yourself. Many of us just can't cope with the practical implications of things falling through, so we ignore the niggles (sometimes with bad consequences). No matter how petty or incoherent your niggle is, get to the bottom of it. As Gavin de Becker puts it in *Protecting the Gift*, his delightfully obsessive book on keeping children safe, when it comes to choosing childcare, 'It's better to look for the storm clouds than to look for the silver lining'. You're never going to be comfortable leaving your baby and going to work if you're not convinced that he's in a safe – and loving – pair of hands.

Pear-shaped plans

Many of us make childcare plans while pregnant that just won't work when we become a mother. 'Before Ella was born I had planned that she'd go to a nursery when I returned to work, when she was six months old,' says Sophie Raworth. 'The nursery we'd chosen was lovely, but a couple of weeks before I was due to go back, I knew I just couldn't leave her there. We eventually found a nanny share instead, and I felt much better about leaving her.' All the books tell you to keep your childcare arrangements simple. But in the real world, many of us end up weepily cobbling things together at the last minute to find an arrangement that we can live with. This, at least, is better than leaving your baby somewhere you feel uneasy about, then spending your working day in a fever of anxiety and guilt.

Your childcare options

Nanny

Cost: around £35,000 a year in inner London for a fully trained, live-in, full-time nanny. Yikes.

How to find one: nanny agencies (try your local phone book), online agencies or look in magazines like *The Lady*.

Pros: good one-to-one care can be reassuring, fun, flexible and nurturing.

Cons: if she leaves suddenly you can be stuffed (this does tend to happen rather a lot), childcare styles can clash, and if she's no good your baby is at her mercy, and hers alone.

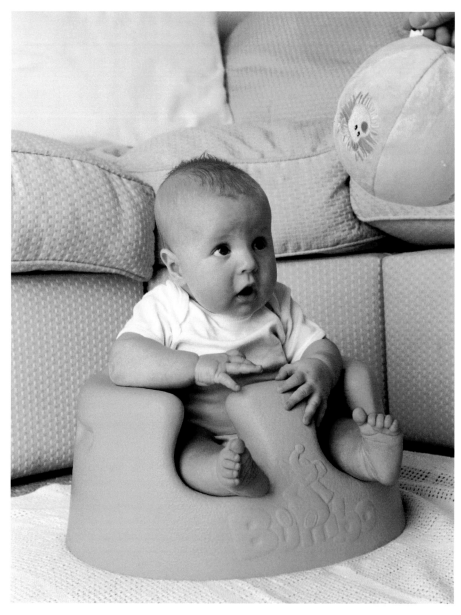

A nanny is expensive, but she will look after your baby in the familiar environment of your own home.

WHAT TO LOOK FOR:

- An NNEB qualification
- References: phone each one individually (don't rely on written ones)
- Her interaction with your baby. Have your baby with you when you interview her. Does she touch him? Speak to him? Ask to cuddle him?
- Your instinct *(see above)*. It's more important than qualifications.

Daycare/nursery

Cost: about £140–£170 a week, but varies widely depending on where you live and what kind of place it is. Expensive does not necessarily mean 'good'.

How to find one: you can get private, community, council and workplace nurseries or daycare – all are registered and inspected by OFSTED. Make a list of all the daycares within a certain radius of your home or work, ask friends and colleagues and try online local mums' groups like www.netmums.co.uk for advice and tips.

Pros: nursery care is reliable and year-round. A good nursery will stimulate your baby's curiosity, learning and social development, and have comforting routines.

Cons: small babies might find a daycare environment overwhelming and may be happier with one-to-one care. Expect quite a few sick days as his immune system learns to cope with all the baby and toddler bugs flying around the building.

WHAT TO LOOK FOR:

- Staff matter more than posh facilities. Do they seem warm and loving towards the children? Are children being cuddled? Encouraged? Smiled at? Played with?
- A good atmosphere. Is it relatively calm, peaceful and under control?
- Happy babies and kids. Do they seem relaxed and playful? How do they interact with the staff? (You're looking for confident, trusting interactions, such as a toddler running to a staff member for comfort.)
- Staff turnover. A reasonably high turnover is the norm for most nurseries, but the really good ones pride themselves on retaining staff, and will tell you this.
- No (or extremely limited) telly. Any nursery that regularly puts babies in high chairs in front of the TV should be instantly crossed off your list.
- Group size. From birth to twenty-three months the legal ratio is three babies to one adult staff member.
- Cleanliness. It says a lot about a nursery, and you don't want your baby getting sick constantly because staff aren't washing their hands, the nappy-changing mat or the toys.

You could also try the Children's Information Service (see **Contacts**).

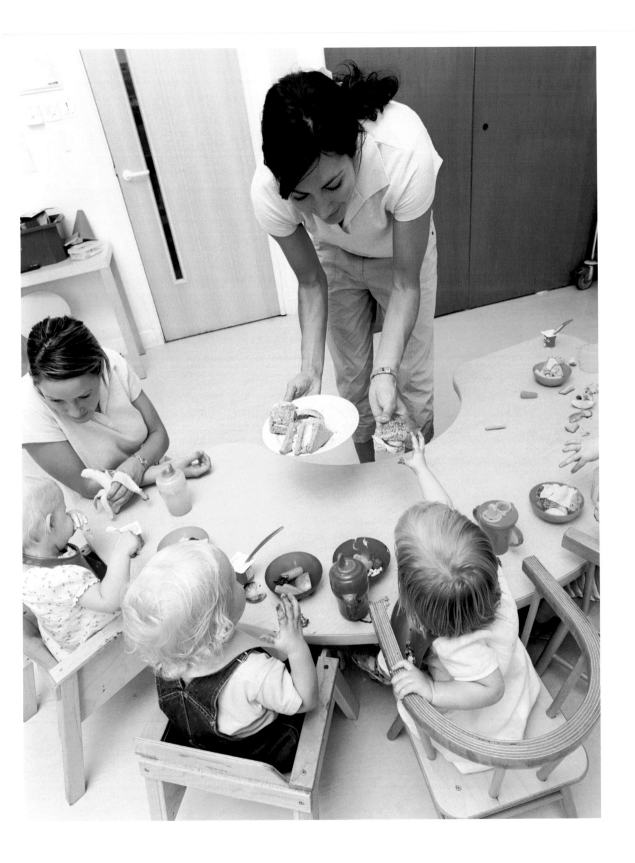

Childminder

Cost: about £90–£140 a week for a full-time place. You'll need to discuss hours and holiday pay.

How to find one: the Children's Information Service is a good place to start (see **Contacts**), as are personal recommendations.

Pros: convenient, more affordable, one-to-one care in a 'normal' home environment, with other children to play with.

Cons: there is no other adult looking on, so you have to be really sure she is kind, competent, loving and safe.

WHAT TO LOOK FOR:

- Registration. She should be registered with your local authority.
- Recommendations by someone you know and trust who shares your standards
- All the things you'd look for in a nanny (except the NNEB)
- You should drop in unexpectedly and see how clean/calm/happy/safe the environment is.

Au pair

Cost: anything from £50–£100 a week, depending on duties. Most will expect to live in and will usually come for anything from three months to a year.

Pros: cheap, and she can be expected to do some housework and evening babysitting.

Cons: she'll probably be young and untrained, may not be used to babies and might be lonely if this is her first time away from home. You may not get to meet her before she comes, and it's debatable how advisable it is to leave an au pair in full-time charge of your baby when you are not in the house (I'd never do it myself).

How to find one: www.greataupairs.co.uk is a good place to start.

WHAT TO LOOK FOR:

- Someone not too young (over eighteen)
- A good grasp of English
- The ability to cook
- A willingness to do housework
- Some previous experience of babies

Relatives

First-time grandparents, if physically capable (in terms of distance and personal fitness), can be the answer to your prayers.

Cost: usually nothing (bar the odd guilt trip).
Pros: a reliable adult who loves your baby just about as much as you do.
Cons: differing approaches/clashes. You have to agree, beforehand, on exactly what's expected: not just the hours (if you're going back to work, you've got to be able to rely on Granny showing up) but the details – there's no good you taking a stand about sweets only to find she's stuffing your baby with lollipops the minute you're out the door.

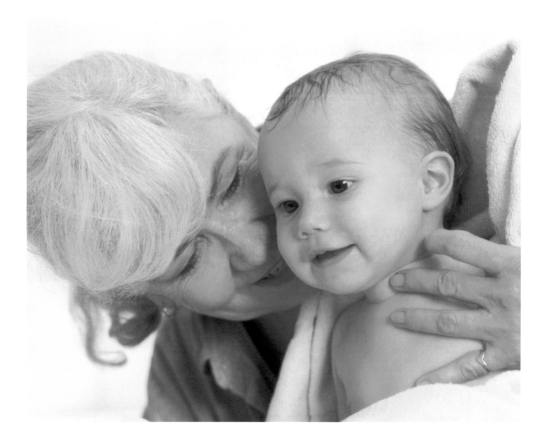

Parent partnership

Some dedicated couples manage to become part-time workers, thereby sharing the childcare – and, we would hope, the domestic tasks – equally. For most of us this is financially and practically a pipe dream, but if it's within your reach, it's got to be worth considering.

Daddy daycare

The at-home dad is no longer a suspect rarity. One third of working mothers cite fathers as the main child-carer while they are at work and, though you might not think it at your average NCT coffee morning, there are now about 155,000 home dads in the UK. Being the only bloke at the swings can make you a bit self-conscious, but it's something most dads quickly get used to. 'On my daily walks I never seemed to see another dad pushing a pram,' says Peter, who was an at-home dad to Amy, now five, for three years. 'I always imagined the other mums were staring at me. In retrospect it was probably our trendy Mamas & Papas pram that they were staring at.' Most fathers, once past any pariah moments, find it all worthwhile. 'I can't say that being a stay-at-home dad was a life-changing event,' says Peter, 'but it was certainly a very enjoyable phase of my life on which I look back with longing in these two-kids, both-working, time-challenged days.'

For other sources of information on where to find childcare, see **Contacts**.

Some ideas for flexible working – for both of you

Your rights

- All parents with a child six years old or under, or a disabled child of eighteen years old or under, have the right to ask their employers for flexible working arrangements, and employers have a legal duty to consider your request seriously – they can only say no if they have a sound business reason.
- The Sex Discrimination Act also says that employers must have a good business reason for refusing to let women work flexibly in order to look after their children.
- You have to put your request in writing and there are various set procedures for this. For more information contact the Maternity Alliance or the Department of Trade and Industry (DTI) interactive guide to help you work out your rights (for details see **Contacts**).

Flexi-hours

Try looking creatively at your working hours. Could you work 7 a.m. to 3 p.m. instead of 9 a.m. to 5 p.m.? Could you go in early one day, come home early another?

Working four days a week

Having one day a week to devote exclusively to your baby can cheer you all up immensely. But there can be pitfalls if you don't work out the small print. 'I felt I was being asked simply to do the same job in less time,' says Jayne, a civil servant, mother of Thoby, three. 'I ended up working evenings and weekends to compensate and felt very stressed.' Make sure you agree with your boss, in writing, what areas of your work you will drop to make your four-day week manageable, and discuss with colleagues how your new working hours will affect them.

Going part-time

If you can arrange (and afford) it, it's worth considering. You get some time for your work, but have less guilt and anxiety about leaving your baby. Many dads are working part-time these days too: in 1986 300,000 men worked part time. By 2001, 1 million did.

Job sharing

It can be hard to arrange and most employers don't want the hassle, but it might be the answer. Have a look at www.flexecutive.co.uk: they have job-searching, a nationwide job-share partner-matching facility and a 'convince my boss' section.

Changing direction completely

Parenthood has certainly spawned many a creative career. I, for one, would not be sitting here now writing books had it not been for my babies. 'I was a real career woman before – very hard-working and successful,' says Jo, an (ex-) financial planner and mother of Josh, five months. 'I thought I would get bored and want to return to work quite soon. I have not been bored and I am leaving my current job and retraining to be a photographer so I am my own boss.'

Back at work: how you might feel

Knackered

Functioning at work – or indeed anywhere – after three hours' sleep is nobody's idea of fun. And if you can barely remember your job title let alone what you're actually supposed to be doing there, it's easy to feel incompetent at first. 'My confidence was at an all-time low,' says Lili, a teacher and mother to Rae, fifteen months. 'By the end of the day

I was flattened, despite ten years' teaching before Rae was born.'
Babies do get bigger, though, and sleep more, so if you can dissemble
your way through the first six months or so you will gradually feel
more human. 'When the twins were one, I realised I was back on
track when I made it through an entire editorial meeting awake,
without the benefit of a double-strength espresso,' says Theresa,
a journalist and mother to Jake and Anya, two. 'There were even
moments when I felt a spark of interest in what was being said.'

Missing your baby

'I hate leaving the baby to go to work,' says Melissa, a writer and
filmmaker. 'I can't bear having to spend so much time away from him.
It breaks my heart really.' It is genuinely hard to get past this, but one
thing to remember is that your baby does not mind who witnesses
his first steps, and he's not going to forget who you are, or think the
nanny is his mother, or prefer the childminder to you. You will always
be his mum and that's huge.

Nothing is going to stop you missing your baby (except possibly
the distraction of work, and simply adapting). Ultimately, if your
working life is really overwhelming you with guilt and loss, it could
be time to explore other options (see page 198).

Guilty

Motherhood, for many working women, can feel like one long guilt
trip with occasional interludes of maternal joy. But dads are not
immune to guilt either. 'I hate leaving my son to go to work,'
says Derek, father of Enrique, eighteen months. 'I commute into
central London and hardly see him during the week. My wife
wants me there more, and I feel that I'm being this old-fashioned,
absentee father – exactly what I set out not to be.'

Once you've weighed up your options and made your choice,
it's worth consciously trying to quell the guilt about the times you're
not there and focus on enjoying your baby when you are there.
Indulging in frenzied 'quality time' to compensate for your absences
won't help either of you. Doing normal stuff – snuggling on the sofa,
tickling, going to the shops together – is more important than
taking your baby to some manufactured developmental activity on a
Saturday out of guilt (unless you want to, of course).

But do try to set aside special time for your baby, time that you'll
spend just being together (without simultaneously trying to catch up
on emails, chat on your mobile or cook a dinner party for eight). You
need devoted, designated baby time – for your sanity, and your baby's.

**HERE ARE FOUR
REASONS NOT TO FEEL
GUILTY ABOUT WORKING:**

1 | No study shows that babies
are damaged if both their
parents work.

2 | Your child will, by and large,
be happier with fulfilled
parents. (Having said this,
if you both work such long
hours that you hardly see
your baby, and when you do
you're too knackered to pay
him much attention, this
comforting adage may
become debatable).

3 | You will enjoy the time you
spend with your baby far
more if you are not beating
yourself up about the times
you're not there.

4 | Your relationship with your
partner is likely to be more
equal and happy if you both
feel fulfilled by your careers.
And, as psychologists never
tire of reminding us, one of
the best things you can do
for your children's long-term
emotional stability is to give
them parents who 'model'
a good relationship.

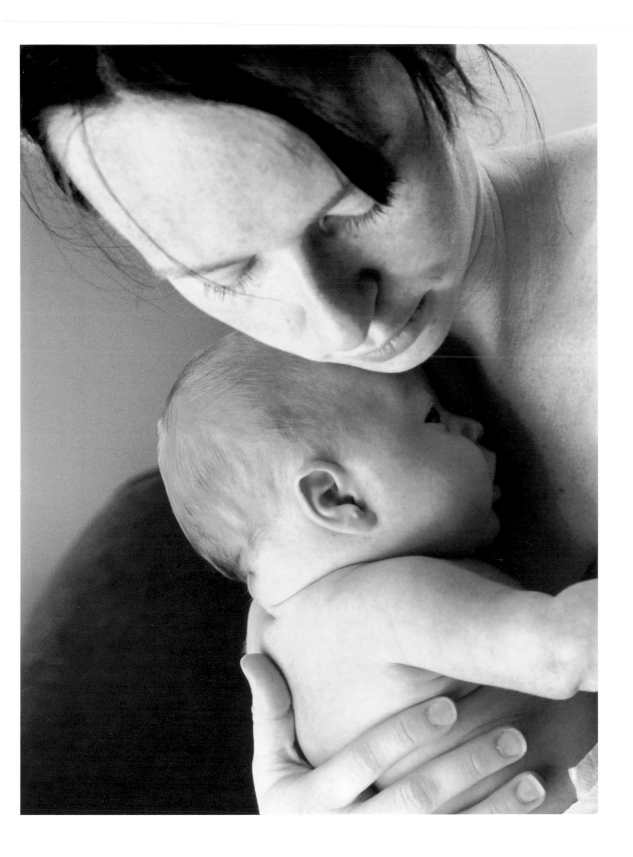

Ambivalence

Ambivalence is pretty much the norm for most working mothers I know (and many working fathers too). I work part-time from home and half the time I'm worrying that I should be downstairs baking my children cookies; the other half I'm fantasising about getting a full-time office job. There's just no easy answer, but if you're basically happy with your work and not desperate to be at home, you're doing marvellously.

Relief

It's a far cry from the image of the career woman weeping over the baby sock she's just plucked from her briefcase, but many new mothers genuinely love going back to work, ambivalence or no ambivalence. 'I went back to work – four days a week – when Milo was three months old,' says TV presenter Emily Maitlis. 'It's never straightforward, but I did feel a huge sigh of relief getting dressed, putting on high heels, jewellery – it felt like my way of saying I was back on track. I've never been someone who stays at home, and I found a real sense of claustrophobia in being at home with a tiny baby.'

Other things that might have changed

Fitting in

Having spent the past several months in grubby sweatpants and gruesome bras, it can be hard to slot yourself back into career-girl mode. 'I saw what sleeplessness does to you,' says Emily Maitlis, 'and I'll admit, I was distinctly worried about how I'd do my job looking terrible in front of a million people.' You may not have to appear before the nation, but squeezing (or failing to squeeze) into your work clothes after having a baby can undermine even the least image-conscious new mother. The top tip here is *shop*: buy yourself a couple of cheap new work outfits in the size you are now, and do not even touch your old ones unless you are 100 per cent confident that you can happily fit into your pre-baby waistbands. It's superficial, I know, but if you look the part you'll feel more confident.

Your ambition

You may find your career has been shunted down your list of priorities in life. Or you may find you just see it all differently now you're a parent. 'I feel more important,' says writer and filmmaker Melissa. 'My life has a purpose and meaning beyond my creativity. I am more ambitious than before because I want my son to be proud of me. I also want to provide for him ... I feel my brain has actually changed in its components somehow – I want to find a way to work that harnesses that.'

Becoming a parent can also give you a tremendous sense of personal security. 'I don't think having a family stops me wanting to push myself to new levels,' says Emily Maitlis, 'but I do know that if I didn't succeed in a certain area, I would feel much more reconciled to that. My family gives me another reason for being alive beyond my work.'

'There is a feeling that people will think you're shirking if you don't keep powering away as if nothing has happened'

Breastfeeding and work

If you don't mind the odd half hour hunched over your breast pump in the loos, this might make you feel more connected to your baby. The idea is that you get your baby used to taking milk from a bottle or cup when you are not there; then, at work, you express milk during the day, keep it cool, bring it home and freeze it. Or you can give your baby formula to drink during the day, but keep breastfeeding in the morning and evening. Contact the National Childbirth Trust, La Leche League or the Association of Breastfeeding Mothers for more information on how to do this.

Fathers and work

Despite all this talk of 'family-friendly' policies, our working culture just isn't on the side of the hands-on dad. Around one in eight fathers in the UK work excessively long hours (sixty hours or more a week), and almost forty per cent work forty-eight hours or more a week. UK fathers, in fact, work the longest hours in Europe.

Recent studies show that dads generally feel discouraged from asking for flexible working hours, taking time off for child-related duties or actually using things like parental leave. There is a feeling that people will think you're shirking if you don't keep powering away as if nothing has happened in your life (despite the cataclysmic fact that is *has*). This pressure is not ideal for babies or their dads. One study from University College London found that babies who did not spend quality time with their fathers – particularly those not regularly bathed by their dads – experienced friendship and relationship difficulties three times above the national average later in life.

If you're prepared to stick your neck out a bit, you may have more bath-time scope than you think. 'I have made it a policy since Joe was born to come home unfashionably early,' says Andrew, who works for a software company. 'I usually make it home by 6.30 and am there to put Joe in his bath, and I read him his story almost every night. At first, I was worried about how this would seem – I used to leave much later – but now people just accept it. I'm on my laptop most evenings, and I make a sneaky effort to send emails at odd hours to "show" I'm working, but I'd rather do it this way than not see my son for most of the week.'

If your work is dispiritingly inflexible, don't panic. Your child's emotional welfare is not all in the bathwater – of course it's not. There are plenty of other ways to be a great father: enjoying what time you do have with your baby is the main one. But it's at least worth seeing if anything can change to reflect the new priority in your life.

Your whacked-out working week

If reduced hours isn't an option, life can get stressful. 'By the time I get home, I'm tired and the baby is tired and grumpy so I miss all of her cheerful times,' says Devon, mother of Ariel, five months. But there are ways to turn this around:

- Juggle your schedule. Try at least to arrange your schedule so that every so often you come home early (even if it means working late and missing bedtime entirely another day). This way you occasionally get a sense of your baby's day before it disintegrates.
- Shift your baby's bedtime. Some couples arrange with the carer that their baby naps later in the afternoon so that bedtime can be pushed back a bit (8 p.m. rather than 7 p.m., with the baby getting up later in the morning). This way they get an extra hour together at the end of each day.

- Prioritise the time you have. Forget phone calls, tidying and laundry when you get home – save all that for when your baby is asleep (unplug the phone and switch off your mobile). And have a big snack late afternoon so you can eat your dinner when your baby is in bed – this way you don't spend precious baby time wrestling with a stir-fry.
- Become supremely organised. One working mother told me that once a month she has a cooking day where she makes four weeks' worth of dinners (not all different …) and freezes them for evening meals.
- Resign yourself to having no life during the week. The upshot of making time for your baby at the end of the day is that evenings disappear – you'll find yourself folding laundry at 10 p.m. then staggering to bed feeling, Where did my life go? The only tip, here, is to hire a weekly babysitter so that you and your partner are forced to go out and have fun one evening out of seven at the very least.

Ultimately, balancing work and baby is, for most of us, an ongoing challenge. You may not feel you've got it right, but just getting something you can live with is a huge achievement.

A quick guide to your rights

Maternity leave

To find out more about what you're entitled to, go to the government's interactive website www.tiger.gov.uk.

- If you were employed while pregnant you are entitled to twenty-six weeks' Ordinary Maternity Leave (OML), no matter how many hours a week you worked or how long you've worked for your employer.
- If you have worked for your employer for at least twenty-six weeks by the fifteenth week before your baby is due, you qualify for Additional Maternity Leave – twenty-six weeks' unpaid leave at the end of your OML.
- You'll either get Maternity Allowance or Statutory Maternity Pay, depending on your working circumstances.
- The earliest you can start your leave is when you are about twenty-nine weeks pregnant. But most new parents say save as much maternity leave as possible for after your baby is born – that's when you're really going to want it.
- When you go back to work after maternity leave your job should, legally, be exactly the same; if that is not reasonably practicable, it should be a suitable job on very similar terms and conditions.

Parental leave

- All new parents qualify for thirteen weeks – per parent, per child – of unpaid leave. You have to take this before your child's fifth birthday, or within five years of adopting.
- For children on Disability Living Allowance (DLA) you can have eighteen weeks' leave, taken before your child is eighteen years old.
- You are also entitled to emergency unpaid leave to make arrangements if your child is ill, hurt in an accident or if there is a sudden problem with care arrangements.

Incidentally, according to the TUC, only four per cent of parents have used parental leave since it was introduced – largely because few of us can afford to take unpaid leave (it has to be taken in blocks of a week).

Paternity leave

- You are entitled to two weeks' paternity leave when your baby is born, for which you will be paid £100 per week (or more, if your company is 'generous').
- You have to have been employed for twenty-six weeks before the fifteenth week before the baby's due date to qualify.
- You can't start your paternity leave until the day your baby is born, and you can only take it in the fifty-six days after the baby is born (if your baby is born early, you can take it up to fifty-six days after your baby's expected date of birth).
- You have to notify your employer that you intend to take paternity leave at the latest during the fifteenth week before the expected week of childbirth.
- Government regulations on maternity and paternity leave and other family entitlements are constantly evolving, so do check out what you're entitled to as soon as you can.

Child benefit

For more sources of information on working rights, see **Contacts**.

- This is a tax-free government handout – currently £16.05 per week – paid to the mother or whoever is responsible for caring for the child (it is not income-related at all), from birth to age sixteen.
- You need to start claiming your child benefit within three months of your baby's birth or you'll lose some of the benefit.

So there you have it: your first year – from the moment you meet your baby to the moment you realise he's a real person (albeit a rather small one) who will cope when you're not there, but will welcome you back with rapture. Parenting is not, then, just about nappies and sleep deprivation and poos and Babygros (though these things are pretty dominant in the first twelve months): it's about the complex business of raising a child, hopefully a happy and healthy one. This is, of course, a bit daunting. But it's also fantastic, because no matter how much you may doubt this at times, it's the one job in the world that you are uniquely qualified to do.

contacts

CHAPTER ONE

Mothercare
t: 0845 330 4030
www.mothercare.com

Babies 'R' Us
t: 0845 7869778
www.babiesrus.co.uk

Mamas & Papas
t: 0870 830 7700
www.mamasandpapas.co.uk

Baby Dan
www.babydan.com

Graco
t: 0870 909 0501
www.graco.co.uk

Bugaboo
t: 0800 587 8265
www.bugaboo.com/uk

Mountain Buggy
t: 01404 815 555
www.mountainbuggy.co.uk

Maclaren
t: 01327 841 300
www.maclaren.co.uk

Phil & Teds
www.philandteds.com

Baby Björn
t: 0870 120 0543
www.babybjorn.com

CHAPTER TWO

BLISS
68 South Lambeth Road
London sw8 1rl
t: 0870 770 0337
e: information@bliss.org.uk
Parent Support Helpline:
Freephone 0500 618140
www.bliss.org.uk

Women's Environmental Network
www.wen.org.uk/nappies

'REAL NAPPY' STARTER KITS

Cotton Bottoms
t: 08707 77 88 99
www.cottonbottoms.co.uk

Eco-babes
t: 01366 387851
www.eco-babes.co.uk

NAPPY LAUNDRY SERVICES

National Association of Nappy Services
www.changeanappy.co.uk

CHAPTER THREE

Association for Post-Natal Illness (APNI)
145 Dawes Road
London sw6 7eb
Helpline: 020 7386 0868
www.apni.org

USEFUL BOOKS

Coping with Post-natal Depression
by Fiona Marshall
(Sheldon Press, UK, 1993)

Antenatal and Postnatal Depression
by Siobhan Curham
(Vermilion, UK, 2000)

*Down Came the Rain: My Journey Through
Postnatal Depression*
by Brooke Shields
(Hyperion, 2005)

CHAPTER FOUR

COT DEATH

Foundation for the Study of Infant Deaths
Artillery House
11–19 Artillery Row
London SW1P 1RT
Helpline: 0870 7870 554
www.sids.org.uk

ONE-PARENT FAMILIES

Gingerbread
Advice line: 0800 018 4318
www.gingerbread.org.uk

One Parent Families
t: 020 7428 5400
www.oneparentfamilies.org.uk

GOOD SLEEP BOOKS

*Healthy Sleep Habits, Happy Child: A Step-by-
step Programme for a Good Night's Sleep*
by Marc Weissbluth
(Vermilion, 2005)

The Good Sleep Guide For You And Your Baby
by Angela Henderson
(Hawthorn Press, 2003)

Solve Your Child's Sleep Problems
by Richard Ferber
(Fireside Books, 1986)

The No-cry Sleep Solution
by Elizabeth Pantley
(Contemporary Books 2002)

CHAPTER FIVE

CRYING HELPLINES

BM CRY-SIS
London WC1N 3XX
t: 08451 228 669
www.cry-sis.org.uk
→ (a national switchboard matches you up
with a local contact who can talk to you)

NSPCC Child Protection Helpline
t: 0808 800 5000

CRANIAL OSTEOPATHY

General Osteopathic Council
t: 020 7357 6655

Sutherland Society
www.cranial.org.uk

COOD BOOKS FOR DEALING WITH
COLICKY/CRYING BABIES:

The Happiest Baby on the Block
by Harvey Karp
(Bantam, 2003)

365 Ways To Calm Your Crying Baby
by Julian Orenstein
(Adams Media Corporation, 1998).
→ Written by an American paediatrician,
this has lots of ideas, particularly
relevant to the first three months

*The Fussy Baby: How To Bring Out The Best In
Your High-Need Child*
by William and Martha Sears.
(La Leche League International, 2002)

CHAPTER SIX

BREASTFEEDING

La Leche League
Helpline: 0845 120 2918
www.laleche.org.uk

National Childbirth Trust (NCT)
Breastfeeding helpline: 0870 444 8708
www.nctpregnancyandbabycare.co.uk

The Breastfeeding Network
Helpline: 0870 900 8787
www.breastfeedingnetwork.org.uk

Association of Breastfeeding Mothers
t: 020 7813 1481
www.abm.me.uk

USEFUL BOOKS

Bestfeeding: Getting Breastfeeding Right for You
by Mary Renfrew, Chloe Fisher,
Suzanne Arms
(Celestial Arts, 2000)

The National Childbirth Trust Book of Breastfeeding
by Mary Smale
(Vermilion, 1992)

OTHER FEEDING ISSUES

Coeliac Society
Helpline: 0870 444 8804

Vegetarian Society
t: 0161 925 2000
www.vegsoc.org
→ The society produces an information leaflet about feeding babies and children

British Nutrition Foundation
t: 020 7404 6504
www.nutrition.org.uk

CHAPTER SEVEN

USEFUL BOOKS

Your Amazing Newborn
by Marshall H Klaus and Phyllis H Klaus
(Da Capo Press, 2000)

The Social Baby: Understanding Babies' Communication from Birth
by Lynne Murray and Liz Andrews
(CP Publishing, 2005)

GROWTH PROBLEMS

Child Growth Foundation
2 Mayfield Avenue
London W4 1PW
t: 020 8994 7625
www.heightmatters.org.uk
→ Information and advice for parents concerned about their child's growth

DISABILITIES GENERALLY

Contact a Family
209-211 City Road
London EC1V 1JN
Helpline: 0808 808 3555
www.cafamily.org.uk
→ Links families of children with special needs through contact lines. Local parent support groups.

Parentability
c/o National Childbirth Trust
Alexandra House
Oldham Terrace
London W3 6NH
t: 0870 444 8707
www.nctpregnancyandbabycare.com
→ A networking part of the National Childbirth Trust for parents of disabled children

Council for Disabled Children Helpline
www.ncb.org.uk/cdc

→ Gives information for parents and details of all organisations offering help with particular disabilities

Are We Nearly There? The Complete Guide to Travelling with Babies, Toddlers and Children by Samantha Gore-Lyons (Virgin Books, 2000)

CHAPTER EIGHT

Talk To Your Baby
National Literacy Trust
Swire House
59 Buckingham Gate
London SW1E 6AJ
t: 020 7828 2435
www.talktoyourbaby.co.uk

Children's Information Services (CIS)
ChildcareLink: 0800 096 02 96
www.childcarelink.gov.uk

→ The CIS will have a list of playgroups and activities in your area.

National Association of Toy & Leisure Libraries
68 Churchway
London NW1 1LT
t: 020 7255 4604
www.natll.org.uk

Sure Start
t: 0870 000 2288
www.surestart.gov.uk

→ Provides information on government support for children, parents and communities and details of local childcare and early-years education.

IDEAS FOR BABY ACTIVITIES AND WAYS TO FIND LOCAL ONES

www.busylittleones.co.uk

TWO GOOD TRAVEL-WITH-BABY WEBSITES

www.babygoes2.com
www.family-travel.co.uk

CHAPTER NINE

Asthma UK
Summit House
70 Wilson Street
London EC2A 2DB
t: 020 7786 4900
Helpline: 0845 7010 203
www.asthma.org.uk

→ Provides information and support for people with asthma, their families and health professionals.

National Eczema Society
Hill House
Highgate Hill
London N19 5NA
t: 020 7281 3553
www.eczema.org

British Skin Foundation
www.britishskinfoundation.org.uk

Meningitis Trust
Fern House
Bath Road
Stroud
Gloucestershire GL5 3TJ
Helpline: 0845 6000 800
www.meningitis-trust.org

Action on Smoking and Health (ASH)
102 Clifton Street
London EC2A 4HW
t: 020 7739 5902
www.ash.org.uk

Child Accident Prevention Trust

t: 020 7608 3828

www.capt.org.uk

→ A great place to go for advice and to learn more about keeping your child safe

NHS Direct

t: 0845 46 47

www.nhsdirect.nhs.uk

→ If you need health information or advice at any time of the day or night, call NHS DIRECT. The website is usually worth a visit for general worries (includes a useful 'body key' tool for working out whether you need to call or not).

Net Doctor

www.netdoctor.co.uk

→ An independent UK-based health website

Action for Sick Children

c/o National Children's Bureau

8 Wakley Street

London EC1V 7QE

t: 020 7843 6444 / 0800 074 4519

www.actionforsickchildren.org

→ Gives information and support to parents and carers

Institute for Complementary Medicine

PO Box 194

London SE16 7QZ

t: 020 7237 5165

www.i-c-m.org.uk

→ Gives information on complementary medicine and referrals to qualified practitioners or helpful organisations

Women's Health

52 Featherstone Street

London EC1Y 8RT

Helpline: 0845 125 5254

www.womenshealthlondon.org.uk

→ Gives information and support on many aspects of women's health and provides a network of individual women who support others with similar health problems

NHS Walk-in Centres

→ are also worth knowing about. They offer fast access to a range of NHS services, including advice and treatment for minor illnesses (coughs, colds, infections) and minor injuries (strains, sprains, cuts). To find out about your local one try www.nhs.uk (click 'No Appointment Needed').

A USEFUL BOOK

Baby and Child Healthcare
by Dr Miriam Stoppard
(Dorling Kindersley, 2001)

CHAPTER TEN

Relate

Herbert Gray College

Little Church Street

Rugby

Warwickshire CV21 3AP

Helpline: 0845 456 1310 / 0845 130 4010

www.relate.org.uk

TO REINFORCE YOUR STATUS AS A MOTHER WHO STILL HAS A BRAIN

www.mumsnet.com

→ Chat and information on all aspects of motherhood

www.badmothersclub.co.uk

→ A bit of fun

A USEFUL BOOK

Baby Shock! Your Relationship Survival Guide
by Elizabeth Martyn
(Vermilion, 2001)

CHAPTER ELEVEN

Children's Information Services (CIS)

ChildcareLink: 0800 096 02 96
www.childcarelink.gov.uk

→ The CIS will have a list of registered childminders, nurseries, playgroups and activities.

Daycare Trust

t: 020 7840 3350
www.daycaretrust.org.uk

→ Gives free information and advice to parents

FOR MORE INFO ON YOUR WORKING RIGHTS

The Maternity Alliance

Unit 3.3
2–6 Northburgh Street
London EC1V OAY
Information Line: 020 7490 7638
www.maternityalliance.org.uk

DTI Interactive Guide

www.tiger.gov.uk

Fathers Direct

Herald House
Lamb's Passage
Bunhill Row
London EC1Y 8TQ
t: 0845 634 1328
www.fathersdirect.com

Working Families

1–3 Berry Street
London EC1V OAA
t: 020 7253 7243
www.workingfamilies.org.uk

→ Tons of info plus legal help and a 'Waving *not* Drowning' resource for parents who have a disabled child and need childcare

www.motheratwork.co.uk

→ Webzine on issues affecting working mothers

www.homedad.org.uk

→ An online support group for stay-at-home dads

THREE WEBSITES WORTH KNOWING ABOUT

www.parentscentre.gov.uk

→ General parenting info

www.babycentre.co.uk

→ General baby info

www.forparentsbyparents.co.uk

→ Parent-to-parent info

index

Many thanks to all the patient health professionals – the midwives, health visitors and doctors – who helped with this book, but especially infant-feeding specialist Sally Inch, GP Dr Louise Hoult, midwife Jenny Smith, emergency-medicine specialist Dr Liza Keating and nutritionist Dr Toni Steer. Thanks also to wise 'baby consultant' Su Moulana, to Sophie Raworth for your support and to Liz Attenborough of Talk to Your Baby at the National Literacy Trust. I am, of course, deeply grateful to all the frazzled new parents who answered questionnaires, subjected themselves to phone interviews, responded to emails, met me in cafés or were otherwise grilled by me when, really, you should have been sleeping – some of you even bravely appear in the photos. And a big thank you to Ben Cowlin for taking those photos so fabulously. A very special thanks to first-time parent Heather Paton who read the proofs while breastfeeding my five-day-old goddaughter Ellie; to Adam Parfitt, Denise Bates and George Capel for making this happen, and, of course, to John for our own first year of parenthood (and the six more since).

A very big thank you to all the mums, dads and babies who took time out from the mayhem to have their photographs taken for this book:

Laurence and Timothy Blackadder, and Ethan
Luc and Dominique Boucher, and Thierry
Natasha and Mark Daynes, and Lucy
Jenny and Justin Fanstone, and Megan
Naomi and Ian Golding, and Katie
Laura and Andy Green, and Harrison
Sophie and Nigel Grice, and William
Ginny and Ken Guest, and Phoebe
Lucy and Mike Healey, and William
Kerry and Oliver Pyle, and Joshua
Peggy Vance, Dharminder Kang, and Jas

The publishers would like to thank Baby Björn, Blooming Marvellous and Mamas & Papas for the kind loan of props for photography, and Sally Inch for her help with the breastfeeding photography.

All photography by Ben Cowlin apart from the following:

2 Imagestate, 10 Imagestate, 22 Imagestate, 24 Getty Images/ Simon Plant, 37 Getty Images/ Ross Whitaker, 42 Getty Images/ Rubberball, 45 Getty Images/ Bob Thomas, 47 Getty Images/ Eisenhut & Mayer, 66 Imagestate, 82 Getty Images/ Sarah M Golonka, 84 Getty Images/ Ghislain & Marie David de Lossy, 98 Imagestate, 101 (centre) From the video 'Breastfeeding - the essentials', Sally Inch/Mark-It TV, 108 Bubbles Photo Library/ Lucy Tizard, 118 Mother & Baby Picture Library/ Ruth Jenkinson, 128 Imagestate, 140 Imagestate, 158 Imagestate, 165 Meningitis Research Foundation, 168 Book Creation, 174 Imagestate, 188 Getty Images/ Mel Yates, 195 Imagestate, 197 Getty Images/ Elyse Lewin